PAIN MANAGEMENT AT THE END OF LIFE

Bridging the Gap Between Knowledge & Practice

EDITED BY
Kenneth J. Doka

Foreword by Kathleen M. Foley, MD
Memorial Sloan-Kettering Cancer Center

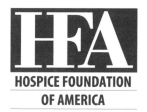

HOSPICE FOUNDATION
OF AMERICA

This book is part of Hospice Foundation of America's *Living With Grief®* series

Supported in part by the Foundation for End-of-Life Care

This book is part of HFA's *Living With Grief* ® series.

Ordering information:

Call Hospice Foundation of America: 800-854-3402

Or write:
Hospice Foundation of America
1621 Connecticut Avenue, NW #300
Washington, DC 20009

Or visit HFA's Web site:
www.hospicefoundation.org

Managing Editor: Amy Tucci
Assistant Managing Editor: Kate Viggiano
Cover Design: Patricia McBride
Typesetting and Design: Pam Page Cullen

Publisher's Cataloging-in-Publication Data
(Prepared by Quality Books Inc.)

> Pain management at the end of life : bridging the gap
> between knowledge and practice / edited by Kenneth J. Doka.
> > p. cm. -- (Living with grief)
> > Includes bibliographical references and index.
> > LCCN 2005937912
> > ISBN-13: 978-1-893349-07-0
> > ISBN-10: 1-893349-07-1
>
> > 1. Pain--Treatment. 2. Palliative treatment.
> > 3. Terminal care.   I. Doka, Kenneth J. II. Hospice
> > II. Hospice Foundation of America.

RB127.P332352 2006   616'.0472
                            QBI05-600224

■ DEDICATION ■

To

Jack D. Gordon

Chairman of the Hospice Foundation of America
1990-2005

For his vision of Hospice
and for the Hospice Foundation of America.

For his wisdom, warmth, and wit
that sustains and inspires us.

May we always meet the standards and example
he so effortlessly set for us.

1922-2005

CONTENTS

SECTION III
PAIN MANAGEMENT AND CONTROL: SOCIETAL ISSUES 209

■ FOREWORD ■

In 1986, the Cancer Unit of the World Health Organization published its first monograph entitled "Cancer Pain Relief." This document set forth a public health approach to the provision of pain relief for terminally ill cancer patients and has served as a model approach to the care of all dying patients. These guidelines were based on the accumulated experience of the international hospice and palliative care movement which had set forth a model care system for dying patients emphasizing the concept of "total pain" and its dimensions: physical, psychological, social, cultural, and the imperative to develop multidisciplinary and interdisciplinary approaches for management. The WHO mandated this translation of knowledge into practice and to use the hospice experience to address the serious epidemic of untreated pain throughout the world. The guiding principle is simple: Provide adequate pain relief to allow dying patients to function as they wish and to die in comfort and with dignity.

Fifty percent of adults with serious life threatening illnesses who died in a hospital experienced moderate to severe pain in the last days of life (SUPPORT, 1995). In the United States numerous surveys document the undertreatment of pain—in dying cancer patients, elderly cancer patients in nursing homes, children with advanced cancer and minorities. These patients could benefit from the use of analgesic regimens based on their intensity of pain. However, significant barriers exist: attitudinal, educational, institutional, political, patient-related and physician-related—and these barriers thwart adequate treatment.

The goal of this book and its associated video teleconference sponsored by the Hospice Foundation of America is to highlight the importance of pain relief and advocate for the better care of patients with pain. This educational initiative focuses on the reality that managing the pain of a patient with advanced illness is the responsibility of health care professionals, patients, families, caregivers and health care policy makers and regulators.

The book is divided into three sections which cover the experience of pain, pain assessment and treatment and the societal issues that impact on inadequate treatment.

Each of the fourteen chapters is authored by experienced professionals who provide an overview of various aspects of pain and its management. A particularly unique feature of this text is an emphasis on the lived experience of patients and families captured from questions asked by patients and families on the Hospice Foundation of America website. The brief discussions in these sections entitled "Beyond Theory" provide concrete, pragmatic information that is so useful in modeling family-centered and patient-centered care. All of the chapters emphasize the need for interdisciplinary teamwork-and again this is modeled by the wide range of expertise of the chapters' authors.

Taking care of the dying patient with pain is a complex process. Healthcare professionals who learn and apply a comprehensive approach to manage the total pain of a dying patient play a vital role in improving the quality of life for both patients and their families. Moreover in their daily work they give voice to the needs of this vulnerable population enhancing their personhood.

Untreated pain wears away at the very personality of the patient and leads families and caregivers bereft that they were not able to provide comfort. These experiences of untreated pain add to the morbidity of the survivor and can influence their own fear of dying in pain. Surveys of the American public on dying repeatedly reveal that fear of pain is a first and overriding concern. This text provides the essential aspects necessary to manage pain in the dying patient. No dying patient should experience uncontrolled pain.

There is now an expansive and documented body of knowledge in treating pain in dying patients. We have international and national guidelines, algorithms for approaches and a vast therapeutic armamentarium. We need to use the knowledge that we have to make pain relief accessible to all dying patients. In doing so, we can honor the legacy of Jack Gordon, who founded the Hospice Foundation of America and served as an untiring and extraordinarily effective voice for advancing hospice care in the United States to ensure pain relief for dying patients.

SUPPORT Principal Investigators. (1995). A controlled trial to improve care for seriously ill hospitalized patients. *JAMA, 274*, 1591-1595

ACKNOWLEDGMENTS

One of my favorite parts of editing or writing a book is the acknowledgments. This offers opportunity to thank all those who have contributed to the task. This year, the task is more difficult as I need to begin by acknowledging the death of Jack Gordon, the founder and chair of the Hospice Foundation of America. Jack's tragic death leaves so many gaps. This teleconference was his vision. Jack was always there to advise and to counsel. I used to joke that I never left a meeting with him without a handful of new things to do. He was even a panelist many times, contributing his legislative and policy insights along with a sharp wit. He will be missed deeply.

Jack would want me to thank the staff of HFA. While the staff is small, they manage to accomplish so much each year. David Abrams, the president of HFA, has kept us focused and offered editorial comments at each stage of the process. Amy Tucci is the managing editor for the book. She has had a gentle and collaborative way of keeping the book on course, and her former career as a journalist has given her a valued overall perspective on this project. Kate Viggiano has ably assisted her. Others in the HFA have provided indirect support, assisting with the foundation's work so the book could reach fruition. These supporters include Sophie Viteri Berman, Robert Lee, Kristen Baker, Jane Pierre, and Bertha Ramirez.

I also thank the administrators and my colleagues at the College of New Rochelle, who create and maintain a warm and supportive environment that allows me to write and edit. I am grateful to so many there, including President Stephen Sweeny, Vice President Joan Bailey, Dean Guy Lometti, and Assistant Dean Marie Ribarich. Mary Whalen and Vera Mezzaucella provide critical administrative assistance. Colleagues at the college as well as those in the Association of Death Education, International Work Group on Dying, Death, and Bereavement, offer ongoing friendship, support, and stimulation.

And, of course, I thank all those in my personal life who offer love and friendship. They keep me grounded—reminding me each day of why this work is so important. My son Michael and his wife Angelina had their second child, Luzelenia or "Lucy" and moved into a new home this year. Perhaps my greatest pleasure is watching them parent. I welcome little Lucy and enjoy observing her toddler brother Kenny as he discovers his world. My godson, Keith Whitehead, continues to succeed in college and to develop into a fine young man, and his relationship with Nicole Martens keeps him grounded. Some of his friends—like Matt Atkins and Kurt Mulligan—remain part of our life.

Other members of my intimate network of family, friends, and neighbors are Kathy Dillon, my sister Dorothy and my brother Franky, and their families, as well as Jim, Karen, and Greg Cassa, Eric Schwarz, Dylan Rieger, Larry Laterza, Ellie Andersen, Paul Kimbal, Don and Carol Ford, Allen and Gail Greenstein, Jim and Mary Millar, Robert and Tracey Levy, Linda and Russell Tellier, Jill Boyer, Terry Webber, Fred and Lisa Amore, Lynn Miller, James Rainbolt, Scott and Lisa Carlson, Tom and Lorraine Carlson, and Don and Lucille Matthews—these people all make life a little more special.

Finally, a big thank you to all the contributing authors who met impossible deadlines with understanding and grace—and with their finished chapters. ■

—Kenneth J. Doka

SECTION I

The Experience of Pain

This book is based on a simple, yet unfortunate, premise: Many people throughout the United States and the world experience far more pain than they should.

Over the past quarter century, the medical profession has made considerable strides in the treatment of pain. In many ways, this progress has been facilitated by the growth of hospice in the United States and other parts of the world. Hospice has pioneered end-of-life palliation, developing a technology for pain management and symptom relief. The result is that people no longer need associate the end of life with excruciating pain.

However, while an effective technology exists for pain management, it is not uniformly available or always applied. There is a gap between knowledge and practice—a gap that this book hopes to address.

The book begins with an overview by JoAnne Reifsynder, PhD, and Douglas J. Weschules, PharmD. Reifsynder and Weschules answer the essential question: Why do individuals experience pain? They describe the pathways of pain, laying a foundation for subsequent chapters on assessment and management. Reifsynder and Weschules remind us that pain is the body's early warning system, alerting us to changes in health.

Next, William M. Lamers, Jr., MD, offers an abbreviated history of pain management. Lamers describes the changing perspectives on pain and the technologies for managing it. He notes that the old ideas of pain as a punishment and asking for relief as a failure of character continue to inhibit effective pain management. Lamers describes two areas in which significant advances have occurred in the management of pain: analgesics and anesthesia. Anesthesiologists continue to be on the cutting edge of palliative care.

"Beyond Theory" is a series of small pieces added to some chapters in the book. These pieces are based on questions asked on the Hospice Foundation of America website (www.hospicefoundation.org). They introduce a real-world perspective and illustrate the concerns of people who are struggling with the experience of pain. The first "Beyond Theory" inquiry concerns complementary pain control therapies, as well as the effect of psychological and spiritual factors on pain. The answer reminds readers of the fact that pain is multifaceted and needs to be treated holistically.

Christine M. Puchalski, MD, further develops this point. Puchalski describes the ways that spiritual and psychological issues can exacerbate pain. Some people make a distinction between *pain* as a physical sensation of discomfort and *suffering* as mental or spiritual anguish. For example, during childbirth, a woman may experience pain without suffering, and anyone can experience suffering without physical pain. However, at the end of life, this distinction becomes relatively meaningless, as mental, physical, and spiritual issues combine to generate pain and suffering. One of the great contributions of Cicely Saunders, the founder of the modern hospice movement, was to recognize the complex nature of end-of-life pain and offer a holistic, team-centered approach to treatment.

In the last chapter in this section, Kenneth J. Doka, PhD, describes the barriers to pain control. He emphasizes that spiritual and cultural factors not only affect the experience of pain; they also can create barriers to effective pain management. Doka's chapter provides a bridge to the next section as he discusses how effective pain management must consider all the factors in the person's environment that might influence how pain is experienced and how it can best be managed. ■

CHAPTER 1

Defining and Responding to Pain: A Priority Across Health Care Settings

Douglas J. Weschules and JoAnne Reifsnyder

Hospice care evolved in the United States in the early 1970s as a spiritually focused grassroots movement in response to gaps in care for persons with advanced illness. As a care model, hospice addresses physical discomfort, emotional and spiritual suffering, social issues, and financial problems. Accordingly, hospice clinicians address pain as a complex phenomenon requiring an interdisciplinary approach. They recognize that individuals' understanding of their pain, fears about illness, concerns about family, and unresolved issues may intensify the perception of physical pain and present a more complex picture for intervention. This essay offers several definitions of pain, explains the sensation and transmission of physical pain, and describes the magnitude of the pain problem in special populations.

THE PERSISTENT PAIN PROBLEM

Despite the enormous and ever-growing body of literature devoted to pain assessment and pain management, pain remains a significant public health issue and continues to be undertreated. Barriers to effective assessment and treatment are especially evident in patients who cannot self-report pain, such as children and cognitively impaired adults, and in cases where there is a language barrier between patient and provider. Many reasons have been cited for this persistent underappreciation of pain, including gaps in clinician education, inadequacy of assessment tools in clinical settings, clinician fears about the use of opioids to treat pain, reluctance among patients to report pain or to accept treatment for their pain, and the historically low priority given to pain management in most treatment settings.

Pain experts McCaffery and Pasero (1999) noted that the accumulated evidence continued to demonstrate that health care systems do not hold clinicians accountable for assessing and relieving pain. However, changes in the regulation and accreditation of health care are fueling necessary improvements in patient care. Many health care settings submit to voluntary review and accreditation by the Joint Commission on Accreditation of Healthcare Organizations (JCAHO). The 2000 JCAHO standards introduced pain management standards that require pain assessment in all patients, documentation of pain assessment, assurance of staff competency, support for appropriate prescriptions, and education for patients and their families about pain and the right to pain relief. Similarly, the American Pain Society Quality of Care Task Force recommends that "all care settings formulate structured, multilevel systems and approaches that ensure prompt recognition and treatment of pain" (Gordon et al., 2005). In addition, advances in state laws on pain policies have had a positive impact on the availability of appropriate drugs and on clinicians' willingness to use them (Gilson, Maurer, & Joranson, 2005).

DEFINING PAIN

Defining pain may appear straightforward to the clinician who does not regularly provide care to patients with cancer pain or chronic pain, or to those in palliative care settings. To a layperson, defining pain may be as easy as reaching for Webster's dictionary. However, attempting to define pain is complicated, especially when trying to encompass all populations, viewpoints, and interpretations. The meaning and connotation of pain and pain-related terminology can vary widely, and the number of terms and the inconsistency in their usage may contribute to difficulties in communication (Turk & Okajuji, as cited in Chapman & Turk, 2001). In recent decades, guidelines for clinicians have presented pain as a completely subjective patient experience. The 1994 publication *Management of Cancer Pain* (Jacox, Car, & Payne, 1994) underscored the need for clinicians to view the patient as the expert about his or her pain and to rely on that individual's self-report as the basis for intervention and evaluation of the effectiveness of the pain management regimen.

Perhaps the most often quoted definition of pain is from the International Association for the Study of Pain (IASP). The IASP defines pain as "an unpleasant sensory and emotional experience associated with actual or potential tissue damage" or is described in terms of such damage (Merskey & Bugduk, 1994). While this scientific definition provides a useful physiologic perspective, it does not fully recognize the interrelationship of emotional, social, spiritual, and other variables that complicate the experience and treatment of pain. The most commonly accepted clinical definition is "pain is whatever the experiencing person says it is, existing whenever the person says it does" (McCaffery, 1968). While somewhat lacking in clinical precision, this definition reflects the subjective and multidimensional nature of pain. Perhaps most germane to the patient approaching the end of life is Dame Cicely Saunders' concept of "total pain," which is a clinical phenomenon that compounds physical and mental distress with social, spiritual, and emotional concerns, demanding a holistic concept of management focused on the individual patient (Clark, 1958, cited in Meldrum, 2003). While each of the three commonly cited definitions is valid and important, none provides us with a universal answer to what appears on the surface to be such a simple question: "What is pain?" Nevertheless, taken together the definitions provide a comprehensive framework for assessment and "measurement" of pain—the necessary antecedents to effective treatment.

PAIN ASSESSMENT

While there is general agreement about the subjectivity of the individual pain experience, there is nevertheless an imperative to measure the intensity, character, and duration of pain across time. When combined with the patient's goals for pain relief, such measurements allow the clinician, patient, and family to evaluate the patient's response to pain interventions and identify exacerbation of pain related to disease progression, failure of the treatment regimen, and changes in patient adherence to the treatment plan. Over the past decade, numerous tools have been developed to quantify what is admittedly a subjective experience in an objective manner. It is important to point out that standardized measures of pain experience are used exclusively for evaluating, aggregating, and reporting the patient's response to treatment—not for making comparisons between patients. Appropriately, such measures are "self-report" tools that provide the patient with a framework for estimating and communicating "how much" and what kind of pain he or she is experiencing. Examples include the Numeric Analog Scale (NAS), Visual Analog Scale (VAS), and category scales such as the Faces Pain Scale (Bieri, Reeve, Champion, Addicoat, & Ziegler, 1990). Yet even when applying these tools to a patient who is willing and able to use them, we still have a difficult time determining which pain is significant and requires intervention, and which does not.

Cleeland suggests that "significant" pain is rated as a 5 or above on a scale of 0-10, as this is the point where patients report substantially more interference with their functioning (Cleeland, 1984; Cleeland et al., 1994). Even with this marker to guide them, clinicians must recognize that to some patients, a score of three is unacceptable. Yet other patients are more willing to cope with a certain level of discomfort—especially when the trade-off may be side effects (real or anticipated) related to analgesic medications. The latter point is typical of an elderly patient who may have one or more comorbidities, such as osteoarthritis, whereas the former example may describe a 30-year-old patient newly diagnosed with breast cancer. Thus, while tools such as the NAS help identify and quantify pain and its severity, they do not define it.

PAIN PERCEPTION AND TRANSMISSION

Pain is a vital adaptive mechanism in normal human physiology. It alerts the individual to the presence of acute and sometimes chronic pathology. Sensory transduction (transmission of painful impulses) in nerves activated by thermal or mechanical energy impinging on specialized nerve endings is known as nociception (Turck & Okijuji, as cited in Chapman & Turk, 2001). The simplest illustration of nociception is banging one's shin or stubbing a toe. The pain appears to be instantaneous, and alerts one to something potentially harmful in the environment—in this example, a misplaced chair or open door! The cascade of events that we recognize as "pain" starts with the conversion of noxious sensory stimuli, such as the banging of a shin on a chair, into an electrical action potential—a process known as transduction (Woolf, 2004). The "noxious stimulus" in the environment must be strong enough for the individual's nervous system to detect its presence. When a stimulus threshold in pain-specific peripheral sensory nerve fibers (i.e., nociceptors) is reached, an action potential is generated.

For most people, a light touch does not reach the "threshold" necessary to elicit a pain response. Stated another way, nociceptors are not spontaneously active and usually respond only to intense stimulation (Woolf, 2004). However, their sensitivity can be altered by local tissue changes such as inflammation or injury. This heightened peripheral sensitivity actually promotes the healing of the injured tissue. Naturally occurring substances, including prostaglandins, leukotrienes, potassium, adenosine triphosphate, glutamate, histamine, and aspartate, can enhance the sensitization of nociceptors to painful stimuli. The transmission of nociceptive action potentials starts at both myelinated (e.g., A delta fiber) and unmyelinated (e.g., C fiber) axons and moves from the periphery to the spinal cord and its dorsal horn. At the dorsal horn, the organization and interpretation of the nociceptive signals mix with other concurrent stimuli and messaging. This process is known as *modulation.*

Melzack and Wall (1965) suggested that their "Gate Control Theory" is activated at this stage. Secondary afferent neurons (i.e., gate cells) calculate the sum of the excitatory and inhibitory signals and interpret what is to be communicated to higher levels of the central nervous system (CNS). Presynaptic and postsynaptic receptors and their corresponding neurotransmitters aid or deter the transmission of these signals. Some of the more significant ones that inhibit this transmission include opioid (mu, kappa, and delta), γ-amino butyric acid, *N*-methyl-D-aspartate, cannabinoid, and α_2 adrenergic. The blockade of one or more sodium- or calcium-channel subtypes also will retard or prevent the transmission of nociceptive or other voltage-gated action potentials across the synapse.

Ascension of nociceptive signaling occurs via the spinothalamic tract of the spinal cord, to the brainstem, hypothalamus, thalamus, limbic system, and cerebral cortex of the brain (Strassels, McNichol, & Suleman, 2005; Woolf, 2004). Pain is perceived at this point on both the sensory and affective levels. The limbic system is responsible for emotional components of pain, such as depression and anxiety. Once this transmission and interpretation is complete, the higher CNS provides signals back to the dorsal horn, nociceptors, and peripheral areas involved in the initial tissue injury, completing the cycle of nociception. To return to our earlier example of banging a shin or stubbing a toe, the nociceptors that are stimulated by the injury transmit information to the spinal cord, which is then communicated to the brain and interpreted, and messages are sent back to the peripheral nerves, observable by the almost instant impulse to pull back the injured body part.

It is at the modulation and translation steps of nociception that most pharmacologic (medications) and nonpharmacologic (cognitive therapies, massage, application of heat or cold, etc.) therapies are applied. However, these therapies are by no means limited to the ascending (afferent) direction of the pathway. Many therapies also inhibit the transmission of nociceptive information during the descending (efferent) part of this loop. Opioids are a good example, as they have antinociceptive functionality in both directions. These receptors and the modulation associated with them, however, are not limited to the dorsal horn. Significant receptor activity, opioid or otherwise, may occur at the peripheral nerve, either helping to raise nociceptive thresholds prior to the transmission stage or helping to reduce signaling after the fact at the local tissue area. This activity can help prevent sensitization and the generation of spontaneous action potentials.

In contrast to nociceptive pain—that is, pain that follows the aforementioned pathway after stimulation of nociceptors—pain can also result from damage to or malfunction of peripheral or central nerves. Commonly referred to as "neuropathic pain," this characteristically spontaneous and often unremitting pain is not associated with the nociceptive stimulus threshold previously described. Neuropathic pain is associated with conditions such as diabetes, herpes zoster (shingles), multiple sclerosis, and "phantom" pain after amputation. Because the mechanism for the pain is different, the treatment modalities differ as well.

This overly simplified description of nociceptive and neuropathic pain is just the tip of the iceberg. Much of what we conceptualize is largely based on theory, and there are still many unanswered questions at every stage of this process. Also, this description provides the reader with a sense of what pain is at the cellular level. It does not illuminate the lived experience of pain from one patient to another.

CLASSIFICATION OF PAIN

As discussed, pain can be characterized as nociceptive or neuropathic, and the physiologic mechanism guides the selection of pharmacologic therapies. Pain can also be classified as either "acute" or "persistent" (chronic) pain, lasting six months or longer. Acute pain most often follows the nociceptive pathway described earlier. Acute pain is a signal that the body has been injured, and individuals experiencing acute pain exhibit similar, observable responses. When a pain stimulus is perceived, the body attempts to adapt to stresses on the organism through the autonomic nervous system (ANS). The ANS regulates body responses that are not under voluntary control, such as heart rate, blood pressure, smooth muscle, visual response (e.g., pupil response), and endocrine response. The ANS is often referred to as the body's "fight or flight" response. Acute pain stimulates the ANS, and increased heart rate, blood pressure, respiration, and perspiration are frequently observed.

When the body is subjected to persistent pain, the ANS response is gradually blunted. Thus patients who experience persistent pain eventually adapt physiologically to the pain and may not "look" as if they are in pain despite profound discomfort. Awareness of this physiologic adaptation to chronic stress has led to more careful assessment of pain and application of the principle that the patient's reports of pain must be believed (Jacox et al., 1994). Further, chronic pain takes a psychological toll. Persistent pain may expand to completely occupy the patient's awareness and can interfere with sleep, nutrition, activity, relationships, and overall quality of life. Persistent pain may be associated with significant fear, profound suffering, depression, and unremitting anxiety.

SPECIAL POPULATIONS

While significant strides have been made over the past half-century toward identification, management, and education related to pain management, it still remains a significant health care problem in the United States, affecting every patient population. Suboptimal treatment of acute pain in the postoperative setting is common in patients with a variety of medical conditions, in minority populations, and across every age group (Gordon et al., 2005; Strassels et al., 2005). Another prominent example of persistently suboptimal treatment is chronic neuropathic pain, which affects more than 2 million Americans (Foley, 2003). Despite the availability and efficacy of antidepressants, anticonvulsants, and opioids to manage pain in these patients, the clinical management of chronic neuropathic pain remains disappointing, controversial, and inadequate (Berger, Dukes, & Oster, 2004; Foley, 2003; Gordon et al., 2005; Woolf, Zeidler, Haglund, Carr, Chaussade, Cucinotta, et al., 2004). Furthermore, while perhaps the most aggressive analgesic prescribing occurs in patients with cancer pain, this population is also undertreated (Miaskowski et al., 2005). This risk of undertreatment is higher for minority groups (Anderson et al., 2002; Cleeland et al., 1994), women (Cleeland et al., 1994), and the elderly (Bernabei et al., 1998; Miaskowski et al., 2005).

The association between age and the undertreatment of pain is not confined to the elderly. For example, it was not that long ago that most clinicians subscribed to the myth that very young infants did not have the neurologic capacity to experience pain. If they did experience pain, they had no memory of it; therefore, infantile pain had no lasting effects. Also, until recently the popular belief held that a child's pain could not be measured accurately (Walco, Cassidy, & Schechter, 1994). As a result of these beliefs, analgesics were used sparingly if at all for infants and children—a practice widely seen as unethical and appalling today. Despite increased interest in pediatric pain management, these patients are still undermedicated compared with the adult population (Ferrell & Rhiner, 1991; Walco et al., 1994). Pain has been reported as one of the most common and distressing symptoms experienced by children with cancer (Collins et al., 2000; 2002); Dougherty & DeBaun, 2003; Story, 1994). Despite the prevalence of pain in this population, Wolfe and colleagues reported that only 27% of children with cancer were successfully treated for pain (Wolfe et al., 2000). Thus, even with the knowledge, technology, and assessment tools to address this important issue, there continues to be a disparity between clinical practice and the need for pain management in the pediatric population (Walco et al., 1994).

We also continue to provide suboptimal analgesia to the elderly— the fastest growing population in the United States. Between 24% and 41% of this population reports *daily pain* (Bernabei et al., 1998; Landi et al., 2001; Won et al., 1999). Furthermore, the prevalence of pain increases with patient age (Bernabei et al., 1998; Landi et al., 2001). The overall prevalence of pain in the elderly population ranges between 49% and 83% (Fox, Raina, & Jadad, 1999). Studies have demonstrated the lack of pain assessment in the elderly (Fujimoto & Coluzzi, 2000), and approximately 25% of patients who do report daily or persistent pain receive no analgesics whatsoever (Bernabei et al., 1998; Won et al., 1999; 2004). When an analgesic is prescribed, the use of inappropriate drugs such as propoxyphene continues (Won et al., 2004), with a significantly higher prevalence occurring in the long-term care setting (Kamal-Bahl, Doshi, Stuart, & Breisacher, 2003).

CONCLUSION

Quantifying the magnitude of this national health care problem across all populations, presentations, and age groups is imperative. For these and many other reasons, education surrounding pain management is still a high priority. The contributing authors of this book are well aware of this continuing need, and all are committed to the management of pain, regardless of specialty, training, focus, or interventions. Our collective wisdom and expertise and the application of our insights by members of the health care profession to patients who are under their care will help to drive both the science and the art of pain management. ■

Douglas J. Weschules, PharmD, BCPS, is the Vice President of Clinical Services for excelleRx, Inc. Dr. Weschules' responsibilities include, but are not limited to: Editor-in-Chief of both the adult and pediatric Medication Use Guidelines (MUGs), member of excelleRx's Research Department, and participant in excelleRx's Compliance and Ethics Committee.

Prior to joining excelleRx, he was a clinical pharmacist for Thomas Jefferson University Hospital, and was primarily responsible for providing and coordinating infusions and related services for patients in long-term care facilities.

Dr. Weschules earned his BS and PharmD from the University of the Sciences in Philadelphia in 1996, and has been with excelleRx since May of 2000. He has gained approximately six years of experience in hospice and palliative care during his employment with excelleRx, and has multiple publications in peer-reviewed journals relating directly to palliative care pharmacotherapy. He also serves as an external reviewer for the peer-reviewed journal Pain Medicine. *Doug achieved his board certification in Pharmacotherapy in 2004.*

JoAnne Reifsnyder PhD, APRN, BC-PCM, is Senior Vice President for Research with Philadelphia-based excelleRx, Inc., a national medication therapy management company serving primarily terminally ill and frail elderly patients in home and community settings. In this role, Dr. Reifsnyder leads a group of clinicians and scientists in a research agenda that includes health services research, technology assessment, a development and validation of clinical decision support tools.

Prior to her current position, Dr. Reifsnyder was a partner in Ethos Consulting group, LLC, a company which she co-founded in 1999. ECG focused on program development, education and training, and research/ evaluation directed at advancing end-of-life care in the United States. Clients included the Office of Academic Affiliations for the Department of Veterans Affairs, Thomas Jefferson University, the Center for Advocacy for the Rights and Interests of the Elderly (CARIE), and ElderCare Ethics Associates.

Previous appointments included Director of Hospice, the VNA of Greater Philadelphia and Director of Patient Services for Samaritan Hospice in NJ. Reifsnyder is currently an adjunct assistant professor and coordinator of the palliative care minor at the University of Pennsylvania School of Nursing. Reifsnyder has numerous publications in peer-reviewed journals, and speaks frequently on topics related to palliative and end-of-life care.

REFERENCES

Anderson, K. O., Richman, S. P., Hurley, J., Palos, G., Valero, V., Mendoza, T. R., et al. (2002). Cancer pain management among underserved minority outpatients: Perceived needs and barriers to optimal control. *Cancer, 94*(8), 2295-2304.

Berger, A., Dukes, E. M., & Oster, G. (2004). Clinical characteristics and economic costs of patients with painful neuropathic disorders. *Journal of Pain, 5,* 143-149.

Bernabei, R., Gambassi, G., Lapane, K., Landi, F., Gatsonis, C., Dunlop, R., et al. (1998). Management of pain in elderly patients with cancer. SAGE study group. Systematic assessment of geriatric drug use via epidemiology. *JAMA, 279*(23), 1877-1882.

Bieri, D., Reeve, R. A., Champion, G. D., Addicoat, L., & Ziegler, J. B. (1990). The Faces Pain Scale for the self-assessment of the severity of pain experienced by children: Development, initial validation, and preliminary investigation for ratio scale properties. *Pain, 41,* 139-150.

Chapman, C. R., & Turk, D. C. (Eds.). (2001). *Bonica's management of pain* (3rd ed.). Philadelphia: Lippincott Williams & Wilkins.

Cleeland, C. S. (1984). The impact of pain on the patient with cancer. *Cancer, 54,* 2635-2641.

Cleeland, C. S., Gonin, R., Hatfield, A. K., Edmonson, J. H., Blum, R. H., Steward, J. A., et al. (1994). Pain and its treatment in outpatients with metastatic cancer. *New England Journal of Medicine, 330*(9), 592-596.

Collins, J. J., Byrnes, M. E., Dunkel, I. J., Lapin, J., Nadel, T., Thaler, H. T., et al. (2000). The measurement of symptoms in children with cancer. *Journal of Pain Symptom Management, 19,* 363-377.

Collins, J. J., Devine, T. D., Dick, G. S., Johnson, E. A., Kilham, H. A., Pinkerton C.R., et al. (2002). The measurement of symptoms in young children with cancer: The validation of the Memorial Assessment Scale in children aged 7-12. *Journal of Pain Symptom Management, 23,* 10-16.

Dougherty, M., & DeBaun, M. R. (2003). Rapid increase of morphine and benzodiazepine usage in the last three days of life in children with cancer is related to neuropathic pain. *Journal of Pediatrics, 142,* 373-376.

Ferrell, B. R., & Rhiner, M. (1991). High-tech comfort: Ethical issues in cancer pain management for the 1990s. *Journal of Clinical Ethics, 2,* 108-115.

Foley, K. M. (2003). Opioids and chronic neuropathic pain (editorial). *New England Journal of Medicine, 348*(13), 1279-1281.

Fox, P. L., Raina, P., & Jadad, A. R. (1999). Prevalence and treatment of pain in older adults in nursing homes and other long-term care institutions: A systematic review. *Canadian Medical Association Journal, 160*(3), 329-333.

Fujimoto, D., & Coluzzi, P. H. (2000). Survey of analgesic use for nonmalignant pain in long-term care facilities in southern California. *Journal of the American Medical Directors Association, 1*(3), 109-113.

Gilson A. M., Maurer M. A., & Joranson D. E. (2005). State policy affecting pain management: recent improvements and the positive impact of regulatory health policies. *Health Policy, 74*(2), 192-204.

Gordon, D. B., Dahl, J. L., Miaskowski, C., McCarberg, B., Todd, K. H., Paice J. A., et al. (2005). American Pain Society recommendation for improving the quality of acute and cancer pain management. American Pain Society Quality of Care Task Force. *Archives of Internal Medicine, 165*, 1574-1580.

Jacox, A., Car, D., & Payne, R. (1994). *Management of cancer pain: Clinical practice guidelines.* Rockville, MD: Agency for Health Care Policy and Research (AHCPR publication no. 94-05592).

Kamal-Bahl, S. J., Doshi, J. A., Stuart, B. C., & Briesacher, B. A. (2003). Propoxyphene use by community-dwelling and institutionalized elderly Medicare beneficiaries. *Journal of the American Geriatrics Society, 51*(8), 1099-1104.

Landi, F., Onder, G., Cesari, M., Gambassi, G, Steel, K., Russo A., Lattanzio F., et al. (2001). Pain management in frail, community-living elderly patients. *Archives of Internal Medicine, 161*(22), 2721-2724.

McCaffery, M. (1968). *Nursing practice theories related to cognition, bodily pain and man-environment interactions.* Los Angeles: UCLA Student's Store.

McCaffery, M., & Pasero C,, (Eds.). (1999). *Pain: Clinical manual,* 2nd ed. St. Louis, MO: Mosby.

Meldrum, M. L. (2003). A capsule history of pain management. *JAMA, 290*(18), 2470-2475.

Melzack, R., & Wall, P. D. (1965). Pain mechanisms: A new theory. *Science, 150*, 971-979.

Merskey, H., Bugduk, N. *Classification of chronic pain. Descriptions of chronic pain syndromes and definitions of pain terms*, 2nd ed. Seattle, WA: IASP Press, 1994. Retrieved November 18, 2005, from www.iasp-pain.org/terms-p.html

Miaskowski, C., Cleary, J., Burney, R., Coyne, P., Finley, R., Foster, R., et al. (2005). *Guideline for the management of cancer pain in adults and children.* Glenview, IL: American Pain Society (APS Clinical Practice Guidelines Series, No. 3).

Storey, P. (1994). Symptom control in advanced cancer. *Seminars in Oncology, 21*, 748-753.

Strassels, S. A., McNichol, E., & Suleman, R. (2005). Postoperative pain management: A practical review, part 1. *American Journal of Health-System Pharmacies, 62*(15), 1904-1916.

Walco, G. A., Cassidy, R. C., & Schechter, N. L. (1994). Pain, hurt, and harm—The ethics of pain control in infants and children. *New England Journal of Medicine, 331*, 541-544.

Wolfe, J. Grier H., Klar, N., Levin, S., Ellenbogen, J., Salem-Schatz, S., et al. (2000). Symptoms and suffering at the end of life in children with cancer. *New England Journal of Medicine, 342*, 326-333.

Won, A., Lapane, K., Gambassi, G., Bernabei, R., Mor, V., & Lipsitz, L. A. (1999). Correlates and management of nonmalignant pain in the nursing home. SAGE Study Group. Systematic assessment of geriatric drug use via epidemiology. *Journal of the American Geriatrics Society, 47*(8), 936-942.

Won, A. B., Lapane, K. L., Vallow, S., Schein, J., Morris, J. N., & Lipsitz, L. A. (2004). Persistent nonmalignant pain and analgesic prescribing patters in elderly nursing home residents. *Journal of the American Geriatrics Society, 52*(6), 867-874.

Woolf, A. D., Zeidler, H., Haglund, U., Carr A., Chaussade S., Cucinotta D., et al. (2004). Musculoskeletal pain in Europe: Its impact and a comparison of population and medical perceptions of treatment in eight European countries. *Annals of the Rheumatic Diseases, 63*, 342-347.

Woolf, C. J. (2004). Pain: Moving from symptom control toward mechanism-specific pharmacologic management. *Annals of Internal Medicine, 140*, 441-451.

CHAPTER 2

A Brief History
of Pain

William M. Lamers, Jr.

INTRODUCTION

In the Judeo-Christian creation story (Gen. 1-3), God created Adam and then created Eve from Adam's rib. They lived in the Garden of Eden, but because they ate the forbidden fruit from the tree of the knowledge of good and evil, God expelled them from the garden and condemned them to a life filled with pain, suffering, and death.

Creation stories have exerted considerable influence on our attitudes about pain and continue to shape lay and professional attitudes toward the relief of suffering. For thousands of years, creation stories such as this one from the Old Testament were offered to explain the constancy of pain in human existence.

Most pain, we now know, can be safely relieved. Surgery, once done in haste to minimize pain, can be conducted safely and painlessly at a more leisurely pace with anesthesia. Childbirth, once inevitably painful, has been considerably freed from the necessary "sorrow" (i.e., pain) predicted in the Bible. The suffering that often accompanies the final stages of diseases such as cancer is coming under increasing control with the proliferation of hospice and palliative care programs and their focus on state-of-the-art pain management.

Yet pain is still a major problem, even in the most advanced countries. In the United States, for example, undertreatment of pain remains a significant challenge. The medical treatment of pain has been so conflated with the social problem of substance abuse that many doctors are reluctant to prescribe analgesic medications for patients with severe, chronic pain. Another factor contributing to undertreatment of pain is the lingering body of misinformation, fears, superstitions, and distorted theology that accumulated over the many centuries before the development of effective pain treatments. In underdeveloped countries, the sheer cost of providing analgesic medications is itself a major public health issue.

This chapter offers an overview of the history of pain, to help the reader understand the reasons behind these persistent fears, as well as the attitudes and misperceptions that continue to interfere with current attempts to provide effective relief of pain. It describes three major advances in pain relief: the development of analgesics, the development of anesthesia, and the emergence of hospice care.

WHAT IS PAIN?

Many people have tried to describe pain. Most have fallen short of the mark. Virginia Woolf captured the futility of trying to describe pain when she wrote:

> English, which can express the thoughts of Hamlet and the
> tragedy of Lear, has no words for the shiver or the headache....
> The merest schoolgirl, when she falls in love, has Shakespeare or
> Keats to speak her mind for her, but let a sufferer try to describe a
> pain to a doctor and language at once runs dry. (Rich, 2005, p. 2)

When asked to describe his pain, an elderly man revealed the multiple dimensions of his pain to Jeanne Quint Benoliel:

> You ask about my pain. That's interesting, because I've been here
> for several months and no one has asked about my pain. What
> pain do you mean? The pain of my life when my daughter died?
> The pain of this disease that's going to kill me? Or the pain I feel
> every day because no one comes to visit me? (Quint, 1967, p. 67)

After considerable debate, the International Association for the Study of Pain (IASP) adopted the following definition of pain in 1986. It contains only the essentials and, while reminiscent of a blind person's description of an elephant, combines complexity with simplicity:

> Pain is an unpleasant sensory and emotional experience with actual or potential tissue damage or expressed in terms of such damage (IASP, 1986, p. 249).

The complexity of this definition reflects the diverse manifestations of pain. Yet it says nothing of the value of pain as a danger signal. The chronic pain associated with progressive disease does not alert the patient to impending danger, as would a painful reaction to heat from an open flame. The IASP definition also says nothing about intensity, site of origin, or duration, as these vary considerably from person to person and from one situation to the next. The definition expresses the dual nature of pain as both an emotional and a sensory experience, and both play important roles in the anticipation, perception, and memory of pain. Tissue damage is mentioned to fix our conception of pain in relation to the body. *Suffering*, a word with which pain is often linked, more properly relates to noncorporeal discomfort, whether or not related to physical discomfort.

Pain and suffering are often combined in vernacular speech in a way that suggests that they are equivalents or frequent companions. Yet, from a medical and psychological standpoint, they have important differences. Pain, more often than not, is a sensation of discomfort, varying in intensity from mild to moderate to severe. Suffering may exist in the absence of physical pain caused by an injury or by damage to or stimulation of some part of the nervous system. It may include an element of physical pain, especially when accompanied by severe, chronic, or recurrent pain, or pain that compromises sleep or physical activity. Suffering commonly includes a troublesome emotional component that may be described in terms frequently associated with anxiety or depression.

UNDERSTANDING PAIN

Pain As Punishment

Throughout history, humans have devised myths to help them understand the nature, and the problem, of pain. The core Judeo-Christian creation story cited above offers an explanation of the origin of the human race. It tells us that pain became an inevitable part of our lives as punishment for the sins of our forebears, Adam and Eve.

The Old Testament also tells us that childbirth is a painful process: "Unto the woman he said, in sorrow shalt thou bring forth children (Gen. 3:16)." Sorrow, we are told, is the Aramaic word for pain.

Every religion and school of philosophy has confronted the problem of pain. Buddhist tradition teaches that all sensations have an element of pain and that pain is due to the frustration of personal desire founded on sensory impressions. Buddhists believe that pain relief can be obtained by following the eightfold path of life. Mohammed taught that anyone suffering from a toothache should lay a finger on the sore spot and recite the 99th verse of the sixth sutra. The Catholic theologian St. Thomas Aquinas believed that "the blessed delight which comes from the contemplation of divine things suffices to reduce bodily pain" (Fülop-Miller, 1938, p. 19).

The persistent belief that pain is a punishment continues to influence our attitudes about pain. A physician friend, Carl Simonton, told me of his mother's saying repeatedly, "Carl, we are put in this world to suffer" (C. Simonton, personal communication, 1992).

Early philosophers also grappled with the problem of pain. Plato believed that pain resulted from a disruption of the four basic elements (earth, air, fire, water), causing a disturbance of the sensitive "soul atoms" that communicate via the nerves to form a tripartite soul. Alcmaeon, by contrast, believed that pain resulted from an unequal balance among the qualities of the elements (moisture, warmth, etc.). Aristotle taught that pain was a passion of the soul. Poseidoneus of Rhodes, a Stoic who entertained Pompey during his own gout attack, believed that pain can be repudiated with reason. Spinoza taught that "suffering ceases to be suffering as soon as we form a clear and concise picture of it" (Fülop-Miller, 1938, p. 19).

Immanuel Kant learned to relieve his own pain through what he called the healing power of intuition. Pascal discovered that if he ignored pain by focusing on mathematical problems and philosophical questions, it would diminish in intensity. These philosophers had learned that it was truly possible to reduce the intensity of pain through distracting techniques that today are called "focused attention," "relaxation," and "avoidance." These techniques worked then and are employed by patients and practitioners today. But they have largely been supplanted by the use of opioids and other chemically formulated analgesic medications.

The frustration our ancestors must have experienced in seeking relief from pain can only be imagined from the extreme means they employed, such as the following folk remedies gathered by Virgilius Ferm:

> Go to a forest and bind the painful part to a tree until the ache is absorbed by the vigorous stem…. To cure a headache, hang the severed head of a buzzard around the neck of the affected person…. Pierce the painful part with a wooden skewer; then bury the skewer in a deep hole in the cellar where neither sun nor moon can penetrate…. Feed the pain to the cattle; burn the pain in a fire; drown the pain in water; bake the pain in gingerbread; hide the pain in an object and palm it off on a beggar (Ferm, 1959, pp. 61-63).

Pain as an Emotion

Before the 19th century, pain was often considered to be an emotion. Numerous explanations of the nature of pain had been offered over the centuries, but the prevailing belief was that pain was an emotion and that if one made a sincere effort, it was possible to reduce or even eliminate pain. Those who were unable to relieve their own pain were seen as having a moral impediment or needing the pain to atone for their sins. Pain was also proof of one's inferior nature or evidence of one's need for punishment. As recently as 1929, a leading medical authority in the United States, Dr. William D. Haggard, Jr., wrote, "Pain, which is the supreme subjective phenomenon of disease, is almost wholly mental" (Fülop-Miller, 1938, p. 19).

This mistaken belief that pain was primarily an emotion was reinforced by common awareness that pain could be intensified or even relieved depending on one's emotional state. Fear and heightened anxiety can intensify the perception of pain, as can anticipation of pain and isolation. Likewise, it has been known for centuries that pain can be reduced by the administration of a chemically inert placebo. Little wonder, then, that the phrase "It's all in your head" has been used to dismiss patients' reports of the intensity of their pain, leaving them to feel that their pain has been undertreated.

Over time, it was learned that the setting or circumstance in which pain was experienced also influenced the intensity of perceived pain. Henry Beecher, who served as a combat surgeon during World War II, compared what he observed in men wounded in combat with patients he had treated during civilian life. He wrote,

> To the civilian, his major surgery was a depressing and
> calamitous event. The soldiers were not unable to feel pain,
> for they complained as vigorously as "normal" men about
> inept vein puncture… [but] I was astonished to find that when
> wounded men were carried into combat hospitals… only one
> out of three complained of enough pain to require morphine.
> The soldiers felt relief, thankful to escape alive from the
> battlefield; even euphoria (Beecher, 1946, pp. 445-454).

What made the difference in the perception of pain? Was it simply the distraction of battle? Was it the result of the increased flow of adrenaline? Was it emotional relief from having escaped death? Today we know that under certain circumstances the body produces its own analgesic substances—endorphins (enkephalins)—that can greatly modify the perception of pain.

Pain as a Physical Phenomenon

The French philosopher René Descartes offered the first explanation of the physical nature of pain during a series of lectures he presented at Oxford University; the lectures were published posthumously in 1664 as De Homine Liber (Foster, Sir M., 1970). Descartes likened the stimulus of pain to a person who pulls on a rope at some part of the body. The rope, in turn, is attached to a bell in the brain. The pain was likened to an alarm system, warning the person that something was wrong and in need of immediate attention.

From anatomical dissections, early physicians came to a rudimentary understanding of how the body works. Modern scientific medicine eventually laid the groundwork that enabled us to grasp the physical basis for pain. We now understand that pain is an innate protective mechanism that has developed within the nervous system to help the organism withdraw from and learn to avoid harmful agents.

Damage to the nervous system can result in pain of various types and intensities. Nerve endings in the skin alert us to our physical environment. Noxious stimuli are generally perceived as painful. Painful sensations are transmitted to the spinal cord by two main types of fibers. A thin, fatty sheath insulates those that are *myelinated*. They conduct stimuli more slowly than the larger *unmyelinated* fibers. Both types of fibers carry painful stimuli to the posterior horn of the spinal cord, from where they emigrate to the *substantia gelatinosa* at the tip of the dorsal horn (gray matter) in the spinal cord. From here they cross to the opposite horn, where they ascend to the thalamus in the brain via the antero-lateral column and are distributed to specific areas of the brain.

Interruption of the spino-thalamic tract impairs pain perception from stimuli applied on the opposite side of body, below the transected antero-lateral column. Pain caused by damage to peripheral nerves is called *causalgia*. Pain from damage to the spinal cord or thalamus is called *central pain*. Central pain and causalgia are also known as *neurogenic pain*.

The balance between large myelinated (fast) fibers and small unmyelinated (slow) fibers is regulated by a gating mechanism that modulates these components. Higher level structures may influence the gating mechanism. Pain may give rise to a number of external manifestations, including but not limited to facial expressions, body movements, guarding (or tensing), crying, screaming, verbalization, avoidance, withdrawal behavior, and contrastimulation (rubbing the skin of the painful area to modify the perception of pain).

MAJOR ADVANCES IN THE TREATMENT OF PAIN

Development of Analgesia

Throughout recorded history, humans have searched for substances to relieve pain. While these searches led to many substances, the opium poppy has been used most often. The opium poppy, the source of morphine and other opioid analgesics, was indigenous to Asia Minor and later was introduced to Greece. The word opium is derived from the Greek word for juice. In the third century BC, Theophrastus was the first to mention poppy juice as an analgesic. He called opium *mekonion*. Another synonym for opium, *thebaicum*, is derived from the Egyptian city of Thebes, where a certain type of opium was produced. The word morphine derives from Morpheus, the Greek god of dreams. In the first century AD, Dioscorides was familiar with the collection and preparation of opium and for preparing "syrup of poppy," called *dia-kodion*. Codeine was the name for the poppy head, from which opioid analgesics were derived. Opium is obtained from milky exudate of the incised unripe seed pod of the poppy plant, *Papaver somniferum*. The milky juice is dried in the air and forms a brown, gummy mass that is powdered to produce opium. There are more than 20 alkaloids in opium, but only 3 have wide clinical use: morphine, codeine, and papaverine (Fülop-Miller, 1938).

Arabian physicians were also familiar with the use of opium, and the Chinese used it primarily to control dysentery because of its constipating effect. By 1500, opium was in use across Europe. The physician Paracelsus, who was mostly identified as German (Fülop-Miller, 1938, p. 24), referred to opium as "the stone of immortality." He was known to compound tincture of opium, called laudanum. Johannes Von Helmont, a noted German physician and a contemporary of Thomas Sydenham, a famous British physician, prescribed opium so frequently that he became know as "Doctor Opiatus." Paregoric (from the Greek word for "soothing") was first compounded from opium by Jacob Le Mort, a chemistry professor at Leyden, in the early 18th century as an elixir for asthma. Sydenham noted,

> Among the remedies which it has pleased Almighty God to give to man to relieve his sufferings, none is so universal and so efficacious as opium (Fülop-Miller, 1938, p. 19).

During the late 18th century, under the Portuguese and later the English, the habit of smoking opium spread throughout China. A mixture of opium and licorice, known as the Brown Mixture because of its color, was introduced in 1814 by Dr. Thomas Barton of Philadelphia. A young German pharmacist in Paderborn named Wilhelm Serturner had isolated and described morphine in 1803, but he did not publish his findings until 1816. In 1832, Frenchman Pierre Robiquet discovered codeine; in 1848, Georg Merck from Germany discovered papaverine.

After these discoveries, the use of pure opioid alkaloids spread rapidly, replacing earlier mixtures of crude opium compounded with other substances. The active alkaloids used as opioid analgesics comprise 25 percent of the weight of opium. There are two distinct chemical classes of opioid analgesics: the phenathrene alkaloids (morphine, codeine, and thebaine) and the benzylisoquinolone alkaloids (papaverine, narcotene, and narceine). Both classes are central to pain management.

Development of Anesthesia

A second major advance in pain management was the development of anesthesia to prevent pain during surgery. Deep sleep has often been likened to a time without pain. In the Old Testament creation story, when God created Eve from the rib of Adam, He caused Adam to fall into a deep sleep (Gen. 2:21). We can imagine that, in this deep sleep, Adam felt no pain from the procedure.

The ancient Egyptians practiced surgery and probably relieved pain through the use of mandragora, an alkaloid of the belladonna group. The Chinese apparently used hashish (*Cannabis indica*) as an analgesic. Pliny, Dioscorides, and Apuleius recommended the use of mandragora before surgery. The Assyrians used a crude method of reducing pain in young boys who were about to be circumcised. They produced pain relief by means of asphyxiation, strangulating the boys until they were unconscious. Italians apparently did same thing to young boys as late as the 17th century (Fülop-Miller, 1938; Melzack, Ronald, & Wall, 1982; Rey, 1995).

The earliest recorded reference to anesthesia dates from St. Hilary of Poliers in De Trinitate in 350 AD:

The soul can be lulled to sleep by drugs, which overcome the pain and produce in the mind a deathlike forgetfulness of its power of sense (Montagu, 1946, p. 113).

Largely because of the pain involved, surgery was not often employed. When it was used, patients were usually premedicated with one of the drugs known to reduce the sensation of pain: opium, belladonna, hemp (cannabis), or alcohol. Further, surgeons worked as fast as possible to minimize the infliction of pain. In the first century AD, the Roman surgeon Aulus Cornelius Celsus wrote:

Resolved to heal the sufferer entrusted to his care, the surgeon must ignore cries and pleadings and do his work regardless of complaints (Fülop-Miller, 1938, p. 7).

Fülop-Miller further relates:

Reports of operations performed in classical times, accounts of those barber-surgeons of the Middle Ages, and the records of modern hospitals before the middle of the Nineteenth Century conjure up scenes of horror. The patient, yelling with fear, was dragged to the operating table, was firmly held by as many as half a dozen stalwarts, feet and hands were tied. Then the surgeon could begin his cruel task, burning with a red-hot iron or cutting into the quivering flesh. The fully conscious patient watched the instruments in the hands of the tormentor, heard the instructions which the surgeon gave to the assistants, each order meaning fresh and yet more intolerable suffering (p. 7).

Major progress to relieve pain during surgery did not occur until after the discovery of volatile gases, including ether, nitrous oxide, and chloroform. In 1540, Valerius Cordus of Germany discovered ether. In 1776, Joseph Priestly of England discovered nitrous oxide. Ether was not used as an anesthetic until 1795, when Richard Pearson of England described the use of inhaled ether to relieve the pain of colic. In the following year, Thomas Beddoes of England described using ether to induce deep sleep. But it was not until 1799 that Humphry Davy of England announced that nitrous oxide could relieve the sense of pain and suggested its use as an anesthetic during surgery. Davy's suggestion was not acted on for 43 more years, until 1842.

In medical circles, ether was considered dangerous in amounts that caused loss of consciousness. In 1824, American Henry Hill Hickman performed surgery on animals "depressed" by carbon dioxide gas. Seven years later, chloroform was discovered. During the 1840s, a number of dentists and physicians showed great interest in the use of gaseous anesthetics to relieve pain during surgical procedures. Part of the impetus came from nonphysicians who used the volatile gases in public demonstrations. During the early 1840s, Gardner Quincy Colton, a chemist and lecturer, gave demonstrations of nitrous oxide ("laughing gas") in New England.

In March 1842, Crawford W. Long of Jefferson, Georgia, removed a small tumor from the neck of a friend who inhaled ether during the procedure. Long did not publish an account of his procedure; therefore, his work did not surface until after William T. G. Morton published the result of his dramatic demonstration of the use of anesthesia to prevent the pain of surgery.

The work of Morton and others in New England in the development of surgical anesthesia changed the history of surgery and, thus, the history of pain. Horace Wells, a Connecticut dentist, attended a demonstration of the effects of nitrous oxide by Gardner Colton in Hartford on December 10, 1844. In that demonstration, a drug clerk named Cooley volunteered to inhale the gas. Cooley became agitated after inhaling the nitrous oxide. Despite the presence of eight strong men in the front row to keep volunteers like Cooley from harming themselves or others, he ran through them and somehow received a cut on his leg. When the effects of the nitrous oxide wore off, Cooley recovered from his daze and noticed the injury to his leg. However, he could recall no pain from the injury.

The following day, Wells underwent a painless dental extraction under nitrous oxide administered by Colton. Several weeks later, Wells went to Massachusetts General Hospital to demonstrate the use of nitrous oxide during a surgical procedure. However, the patient awakened too soon, screaming in pain, and the use of nitrous oxide was discredited.

In 1846, ether was introduced as an anesthetic. William Morton, a dental associate of Wells, had entered Harvard Medical School. In order to defray the expense of his education, he continued his dental practice. Morton's chemistry professor told him that sulfuric ether would work better than ethyl ether. Morton persuaded J. C. Warren, professor of surgery at Harvard, to demonstrate the use of ether as an anesthetic in surgery. The date was October 16, 1846. The patient's name was Gilbert Abbott. When Morton failed to appear in the surgical amphitheater at the appointed time to deliver the anesthetic, Warren, dressed in formal morning clothes, appeared ready to proceed without benefit of anesthesia.

When Morton appeared, Warren remarked, "Well, sir, *your* patient is ready." Morton administered ether anesthesia to Abbott and, turning to Warren, said, "Doctor, your patient is ready." Upon completion of the surgical procedure, Warren said to the audience, "Gentlemen; this is no humbug!" The dean of the medical school, Henry Jacob Bigelow, said, "I have seen something today that will go around the world." Years later, Bigelow wrote the inscription that is engraved on Morton's tomb:

> Inventor and Revealer of Anaesthetic Inhalation.
> Before Whom, in All Time, Surgery was Agony.
> By Whom Pain in Surgery Was Averted and Annulled.
> Since Whom Science Has Control of Pain.

In recent years, techniques derived from surgical anesthesia have been used in a variety of other ways to manage patients' pain. Anesthesia professionals are playing increasing roles beyond the surgical setting in hospital pain services and as consultants to hospice and palliative care programs to address pain that cannot be adequately relieved with analgesics alone. Techniques such as nerve blocks, intraspinal (intrathecal and epidural) pharmacology, cordotomy, and neuro-destructive procedures are among the techniques used in this context (Reisfield, 2001).

Hospice and Pain Management

A third major advance in pain management began with the emergence of hospice as an organization dedicated to allowing terminally ill patients to live in dignity and comfort until their death. Since the opening of St. Christopher's Hospice in London in 1967, many health care workers have developed an interest in providing improved care to persons with advanced and incurable illness. Without its steadfast emphasis on pain management, the international hospice movement likely would not have gained worldwide acceptance.

The poor level of conventional medical care for dying persons, especially inadequate pain relief, led John Hinton, an English physician, to proclaim:

> We emerge deserving of little credit; we who are capable of
> ignoring the conditions that make muted people suffer. The
> dissatisfied dead cannot noise abroad the negligence they have
> experienced (Hinton, 1972, excerpted from a letter).

The failure to treat pain in dying persons was only part of the huge problem of lack of attention to their needs. Aring characterized the problem many physicians experienced in caring for dying patients:

> The physician, unaware of his personal feelings about death and
> dying, by the same token enables them to interfere with his effec-
> tive treatment of patients. On one hand, indifference has resulted
> in undertreatment or neglect and, on the other, in overtreatment
> and the officious striving to keep alive (Aring, 1969, p. 160).

Cicely Saunders, founder of St. Christopher's Hospice and of the modern hospice movement, thoroughly researched the chronic and sometimes severe pain that accompanies some end-stage conditions. She found that severe, chronic pain never occurs by itself but is always accompanied by other phenomena, including anxiety, depression, fear, insomnia, anorexia, frustration, anger, self-recrimination, and thoughts of suicide. Severe, chronic pain incorporates the recollection of past pain, the sensation of currently experienced pain, and the anticipation of pain yet to come.

All these factors, taken together, contribute to a lowering of the pain threshold so that even usually tolerated sounds and bright lights can inten-sify the perception of pain. Saunders, who incorporated these factors into her concept of "total pain," emphasized that symptom management and pain control were the essence of the good palliative care necessary to allow dying persons to live their final days in reasonable comfort.

The worldwide hospice movement has been noteworthy in advocating the use of opioid analgesics to manage severe, chronic pain. St. Christopher's initially advocated Brompton Mixture (heroin, cocaine, chloroform water, a phenothiazine, and alcohol) to be administered every 4 hours in a dose sufficient to relieve pain. As heroin could not be prescribed in the United States and morphine was as effective as heroin (the other ingredients in Brompton were essentially superfluous to pain relief), oral morphine solution gained wide acceptance in this country as the foundation of hospice pain management.

Over time, other opioid analgesics, including extended-relief preparations and transdermal applications, have gained wide acceptance. Hospice professionals have also learned to monitor and manage the three most common side effects of opioid analgesics: drowsiness (usually transient), nausea and vomiting (usually transient), and constipation (persistent and in need of continuing attention). Problems associated with the recreational use of opioids (tolerance, addiction, overdose) are rarely observed in patients treated for pain and are not contraindications to the careful prescribing and administration of opioids in hospice care.

Hospices pioneered much of the foundational research on pain control with opioids. They also emphasized two other core ideas. First, since pain and suffering are multifaceted, pain management must be holistic—encompassing the physical but also the psychological, social, and spiritual domains. Second, such an approach necessitates a different organization of care. The hierarchical organization of traditional medical care needs to be replaced by a truly interdisciplinary team approach.

BARRIERS TO HOSPICE

Change does not come easily. Hospice care and excellent pain management have not been embraced as rapidly as advocates believe they should be. Despite the fact that almost a million persons in the United States alone will receive hospice care in 2005, a larger number of dying persons who would benefit from such care will not receive it. The following are some of the factors inhibiting wider use of hospice care:

- Physician reluctance to "admit defeat."
- Physician reluctance to turn their patients' medical care over to someone else.

- Economics of patients not yet eligible for the Medicare hospice benefit.

- Lack of physician education about hospice care.

Other problems limit the wider availability of excellent pain management and contribute to the widespread problem of undertreatment of pain:

- Physicians fear accidental or intentional overdose by patients.

- Physicians fear diversion of opioids to illicit use.

- Physicians fear censure or loss of their license to practice medicine for prescribing opioids or criminal prosecution for violating federal prescribing statutes.

- Physicians fear the development of addiction in patients given opioids.

- Physicians fear the development of tolerance to opioids.

- Physicians are poorly trained to manage severe, chronic pain.

- Patients are afraid to take opioid medications.

- Some patients still believe there is a value in suffering or that suffering is punishment for their sins.

- Some patients experience side effects that, left untreated, discourage them.

- Some patients cannot afford the medications that would relieve their pain.

- Some patients perceive a negative societal stigma to using opioids.

- The lay public lacks accurate information about opioid analgesics.

- A just say no mentality inhibits the proper use of opioid analgesics.

- Physicians tend to underestimate the intensity of their patients' pain.

Recently, there has been a movement to extend the principles of hospice care to patients who do not have a time-limited prognosis (currently a prerequisite for hospice enrollment). This approach, called "palliative care," is designed to provide other patients with the pain management and symptom relief characteristic of hospice care. The word *palliation* is derived from the Latin word for "cloak" and implies a "covering over" of symptoms when cure is not possible. Many hospitals have begun to develop palliative care consultation teams and even dedicated palliative care units, where special attention is paid to symptom management and pain relief.

CONCLUSION

Despite advances in its management, pain is still a major worldwide health problem. Even with the availability of excellent analgesics in developed countries such as the United States, undertreatment of pain of all sorts remains a major challenge. Some of the persistent fears, inappropriate attitudes, and misperceptions that interfere with our attempts to relieve pain have been described.

In some underdeveloped countries, pain appears to be an insoluble problem from an economic standpoint. We know how to provide safe relief for severe, chronic pain, and the medications are available. But there is no adequate health care delivery system and no money to buy the drugs that could be used to relieve pain. McCleane has pinpointed the great challenge that lies before us:

> But has our ability to treat pain actually improved? An emphatic yes to this question can be given by those living in the so called "developed" world. But could such a positive response be given by those living in more underdeveloped areas? Most newly released drugs come with such a hefty price tag that their use would be prohibitively expensive in many areas of the world (McCleane, 2005, p. 1). ■

William M. Lamers, Jr., MD, is Medical Consultant to the Hospice Foundation of America. Following his training in medicine, psychiatry and child psychiatry, and service in the U.S. Navy Medical Corps during the Vietnam war, Dr. Lamers joined the clinical faculty of the University of California, San Francisco, where he taught medical students in the Department of Ambulatory and Community Medicine. During the early 1970s, Dr. Lamers developed Hospice of Marin, one of the first home care hospice programs in the United States. He served as Chair of Standards and Accreditation Committee of the National Hospice Organization (now NHPCO). He is past-president of the International Work Group on Death, Dying and Bereavement (IWG). Dr. Lamers has taught widely in the United States and many foreign countries. He has contributed numerous articles and chapters to the literature on subjects including hospice, grief, bioethics, poetry, and pain management to the development of community support for caregivers. He has served as medical-legal expert witness in litigation related to dying, death, burial, cremation, organ donation, and murder. He is on the editorial boards of several professional journals in the field of pain management. He lives in southern California.

REFERENCES

Aring, C. D. (1969). *The understanding physician: Writings of Charles D. Aring, M.D.* Detroit: Wayne State University Press.

Beecher, H. K. (1946). Pain in men wounded in battle. *Bulletin of U.S. Army Medical Department, 5*, 445-454.

Gen. 2:21, King James Bible.

Gen. 3:16, King James Bible.

Ferm, V. (1959). *A brief dictionary of American superstitions.* New York: Philosophical Library.

Foster, Sir M. (1970). *Lectures on the history of physiology during the sixteenth, seventeenth, and eighteenth centuries.* New York: Dover Publications.

Fülop-Miller, R. (1938). *Triumph over pain.* London: Hamish-Hamilton, Ltd.

Haggard, W. (1929). *Devils, drugs and doctors.* New York: Blue Ribbon Books.

Hinton, J. (1972). *Dying.* Harmondsworth, England: Penguin.

International Association for the Study of Pain (IASP) Subcommittee on Taxonomy. (1978). Pain terms: A list with definitions and notes on usage. *Pain, 8,* 249-252.

McCleane, G. (2005). Editorial. *Journal of Neuropathic Pain and Symptom Palliation, 1*(2), 1-2.

Montagu, M. F. A. (1946). Fourth century reference to anesthesia. *Bulletin of the History of Medicine, 19,* 113-114.

Quint, J. C. (1967). *The Nurse and the dying patient.* New York: MacMillan.

Reisfield, G. (2001, May). Pain management at the end of life (the hospice patient). *Jacksonville Medicine.* Retrieved July 14, 2005, from www.dcmsonline.org/jax-medicine/2001journals/May2001/paincontrol.htm

Rich, B. A. (2005, Spring). The humanistic dimensions of pain and suffering in the clinical setting. *Practical Bioethics, 1*(2), 1-2.

Sydenham, T. (1680). In Rey, Roselyne [Ed.]. *The History of Pain* (1995, p. 65). Cambridge, Mass.: Harvard University Press. Translated by Louise Elliott Wallace, J. A., Cadden & S. W. Cadden.

COMMON MYTHS ABOUT PAIN

Myth: *"Dying is always painful."*
Many people die without experiencing pain. If pain does occur, it can be relieved safely and rapidly.

Myth: *"Some kinds of pain can't be relieved."*
There are some types of pain that require "multi-modality" (combined approaches) pain relief. Recent advances in analgesia ensure that all pain can be relieved by using commonly available medications and/or a combination of approaches that may include chemotherapy, radiation therapy, nerve block, physical therapies, and whatever else is appropriate.

Myth: *"Pain medications always cause heavy sedation."*
Most people with severe, chronic pain have been unable to sleep because of their pain. The opioid analgesics (morphine, codeine, etc.) produce initial sedation (usually about 24 hours) that allows patients to catch up on their lost sleep. With continuing doses of medication they are able to carry on normal mental activities. Sedation often occurs because of other drugs, such as anti-anxiety agents and tranquilizers that have been prescribed for other reasons.

Myth: *"It is best to save the stronger pain relievers until the very end."*
If pain is not relieved by the lesser strength analgesics (aspirin, NSAIDs, codeine, hydrocodone, etc.) then it is best to change to a stronger analgesic to bring the pain under continuing (24-hour) control. Pain that is only partially or occasionally controlled tends to increase in severity. This leads to two mistaken assumptions: the patient mistakenly fears that the pain is so severe that it can never be controlled; the doctor mistakenly believes that the patient is becoming addicted or is developing tolerance to the analgesic medication. In most cases, an adequate dose of a stronger analgesic (e.g., morphine) prescribed on a regular basis usually brings the pain under control.

continued

Myth: *"Patients often develop tolerance to pain medications like morphine."*

When morphine and other opioid analgesics are prescribed for the management of pain, the dose is sometimes raised to be sure that pain is well-controlled 24 hours a day, 7 days a week. Opioids given to relieve pain generally do not lead to the development of tolerance. As a disease, like cancer, progresses, more opioid may be needed to control the pain on a continuing basis.

Myth: *"Once you start pain medicines, you always have to increase the dose."*

In fact, the converse is true. Once pain is under control and the dose of opioid held at a steady level for several days, the dose of opioid analgesic can be lowered without the pain recurring. Levels of opioid can be raised safely as needed to control increasing pain. Also, the dose can be lowered gradually if pain has been controlled on the same dose for several days. This change in dose to meet patient needs is known as "titration." The fact that the dose of opioid can be lowered once pain is controlled is one of the paradoxes of treating severe, chronic pain.

Myth: *"To get good pain relief, you have to take injections."*

Until the mid-1970s it was believed that morphine was not an effective analgesic when administered by mouth, so it was universally administered by injection. We now know that morphine is effective when given by mouth or even by suppository. Patients generally do not like injections, as they are painful in themselves. There are several excellent long-acting opioid analgesic preparations. Morphine and related opioids are available that control pain for 12 hours when used on a regular basis twice daily. Other long-acting opioid preparations available for trans-dermal (through the skin) delivery are available with a 72-hour (3-day) period of action.

Myth: *"Pain medications always lead to addiction."*

When prescribed on a regular basis in a dose sufficient to relieve pain, there is no empirically based evidence that opioids lead to addition.

Myth: *"Withdrawal is always a problem with pain medications."*

When prescribed for managing severe, chronic pain there is no problem discontinuing the dose once pain is controlled. Withdrawal from the opioid analgesics is not a life-threatening condition as is withdrawal from a number of other commonly prescribed medications, such as barbiturates. The symptoms of withdrawal from opioids are generally mild and fairly easy to manage with commonly available medications. Many patients who receive opioids for severe pain have had their dose adjusted down without experiencing any withdrawal symptoms.

Myth: *"Enduring pain and suffering can enhance one's character."*

This myth developed in the years before we learned to provide excellent pain management, but is not appropriate today. Suffering does not enhance character or earn people a higher place in the life hereafter; it merely brings about a miserable life, a horrible death, and needless anguish in all who see helpless dying people suffer.

Myth: *"Once you start taking morphine, the end is always near."*

Morphine does not initiate the final phase of life or lead directly to death. Morphine provides not only relief of severe, chronic pain; it also provides a sense of comfort. It makes breathing easier. It lets the patient relax and sleep. It does not cloud consciousness or lead to death. Morphine does not kill.

Myth: *"Pain is a solitary phenomenon."*

Severe chronic pain never occurs alone, but is usually accompanied by a number of other symptoms including (but not limited to) anxiety, depression, fearfulness, insomnia, anorexia (loss of appetite), withdrawal and thoughts of suicide. All of these symptoms are compounded with memories of pain already experienced, currently perceived pain, and anticipation of more pain yet to come. Unmanaged (or inadequately managed) severe, chronic pain is a complex problem that needlessly aggravates the symptoms of the underlying disease.

continued

Myth: *"Heroin is needed to provide excellent pain control."*
Heroin is a derivative of morphine that is more soluble in water than morphine and therefore passes from the blood to the brain more rapidly, thus affording the "rush' or "high" desired by intravenous drug abusers. Morphine has a longer period of action. It can be safely taken by mouth. New preparations for sustained release make it possible to obtain excellent relief when taken by mouth only twice daily.

Myth: *"People have to be in a hospital to receive effective pain management."*
It is easier to provide safe, effective relief of severe chronic pain at home than it is in the average hospital. There are fewer medication errors when there is only one patient to receive medications and no other patient emergencies to interrupt the care. Accurate messages regarding pain management can be shared on a regular basis by means of a "Comfort Control Chart" on which the patient indicates the level of pain relief by using numbers (0 to 10) to let the doctor know the adequacy of pain management.

Source: Hospice Foundation of America

■ CHAPTER 3 ■

Spirituality in the Care of the Aging and Dying

Christina M. Puchalski

INTRODUCTION

Aging and dying are integral and normal parts of living; in our society, however, they are treated as something to be avoided at all costs. While there have been remarkable improvements in the care of chronically ill and dying patients, much remains to be done to ensure that all people are treated with dignity and respect.

People have an inherent value as human beings, whether they are young or old, healthy or ill, in the prime of life or dying. Yet, our society and our health care systems do not yet reflect that. Television shows, media of all kinds, and innovations in medication and plastic surgery reflect the philosophy that we must try to stay young and active as long as possible. They support physical transformation to maintain youth in both actions and looks. Aging and dying are not taken into consideration in society's quest for the fountain of youth.

This philosophy is reflected in our health care system. Research dollars are allocated toward cures and treatments that prolong life, some of which pay only minimal attention to the quality of that life. Health insurance coverage benefits the young and healthy. Those over 65 are rejected by some plans and by physicians who cannot afford to deal with the increasingly burdensome Medicare system of reimbursement. Thus, as people age and deal with severe illness and with dying, they often feel less of a person than when they were younger and healthier. All too often, people die in hospitals or nursing homes, alone and burdened with unnecessary treatment; treatment they would have refused if they had had the chance to talk about their choices with their physicians long before the deathbed scene. Aging and dying people are not listened to. Their wishes, dreams, and fears often go unheeded, no matter how much they want to share them with their loved ones and with health care professionals.

Aging and dying are part of life. They should be honored and valued and given their proper place in the large scheme of life, just as other stages of living are. In some cultures, the old and dying are given the highest place of honor. These are people who have given of themselves for many years, have experienced many facets of life, and now are seen as the great teachers and honored members of society. In some societies, reaching old age or the time of dying is viewed as an accomplishment, not something shameful. If we could change our own society's outlook on aging and dying, we could transform the care of the elderly and the seriously ill in a major way. Aging and dying well would be perceived as something to aspire to and to do with grace and dignity.

SPIRITUALITY IS ESSENTIAL TO HEALTH CARE AND LIVING

One way to transform the way our society and our health care system view aging and dying is to recognize that spirituality is essential to health care and, in fact, to life itself. Spirituality can be defined as the essence of our humanity (Frankl, 1984). It is the part of us that energizes us to move forward in our lives, to find meaning and purpose, and to connect with God/Divine and others. Spirituality is the source of inner healing and strength in each person; it is both the life-giving force and the force that allows us to accept aging and our eventual death. As healthy young people, we may accept a belief system with little self-reflection or examination; our belief system may come from traditional values passed on by parents and teachers. As we face life's difficulties—such as illness and the loss of dreams or loved ones—we may question our basic beliefs. Questions such as "Why me?" and "Why now?" can trigger a deep spiritual quest into what ultimately gives meaning and purpose to our lives. As we age and/or face our own death, we can no longer defer growth and introspection to a later time. In the nakedness of dying, we face ourselves in the most honest and genuine way. It is there that spiritual transformation may occur.

James Fowler (1981) proposes six stages of faith development. In the sixth and final stage, which he calls *universalizing*, older adults begin to search for universal values such as justice and unconditional love. Self-oriented values such as self-preservation no longer hold primary importance. One can understand why aging and dying people are revered in many cultures, for it is in these profound phases of life that spiritual wisdom can be acquired.

Dying may be the ultimate spiritual challenge. Death is an unknown. The mystery surrounding life and death can frighten people, as we cling to certitude. Spiritual journeys can be shaped and challenged by facing this uncertainty and mystery. Our previous beliefs—in God's power, that prayer brings cures, that the community can help overcome suffering, that science has all the answers—might not help us in the face of our inevitable death. We may give up entirely on our beliefs, or we might be spurred to evaluate our beliefs on a deeper level. We might integrate religious dogma and beliefs into less definable spiritual beliefs. Chandler (1999) distinguishes spiritual journeys from religious beliefs in that the former "involve us in the mystery of experiencing the holy, the mysterious" (p. 65). Is it possible to have meaning and purpose, an implied knowledge of self, in the midst of mystery and unknowing? Meaning can be found in many places—in relationships, in God, in the illness itself, in service to others, in love. But even the meaning we find in these places may be surrounded in mystery. As Reinhold Niebuhr wrote, "Thus, wisdom about our destiny is dependent upon a humble recognition of the limits of our knowledge and our power. Our most reliable understanding is the fruit of 'grace,' in which faith completes our ignorance without pretending to possess its certainties as knowledge" (Brown, 1986, p. 66).

As one who cares for the chronically ill and dying, I have shared others' challenges and spiritual journeys, and witnessed tremendous sadness as well as joy. People who have struggled with suffering and have managed to find some meaning for themselves in the midst of that suffering may not always be joyful and blissful, but they often are at peace and content with their lives and with themselves. They see themselves with clarity, honesty, and love. This is, as Fowler writes, the highest form of spiritual development. Imagine a television show that portrays the wisdom of those who face aging, serious illness, and dying rather than a show about people who have had extensive cosmetic surgery to try to regain the faces and physiques they had 20 years ago. I believe the result would be to honor what is critical to all people: their spirituality.

SPIRITUAL CARE OF THE AGING AND THE DYING

Aging and dying should be as natural an experience as birth. It should be a time when people find meaning in their suffering and when all the dimensions of their experience are addressed by their caregivers. These dimensions, from the hospice model developed by Cicely Saunders, are as follows (Wald, 1986):

- the physical (pain and symptom control);
- the psychological (anxiety and depression);
- the social (feeling cut off from friends and family, feeling too fatigued to engage in social activities); and
- the spiritual.

It is our responsibility to listen to people as they struggle with their dying. We need to be willing to listen to their anxieties, their fears, their unresolved conflicts, their hopes, and their despair. If people are stuck in despair, they will suffer deeply. It is through spirituality that people become unstuck from despair. Viktor Frankl wrote that man is not destroyed by suffering; he is destroyed by suffering without meaning. Spirituality helps give meaning to people's suffering. It helps people find hope in the midst of despair. We, as caregivers, need to engage with our patients on the spiritual level.

The fact that spirituality is of primary importance to the dying person is recognized by many experts and by our patients themselves. A Gallup International Institute survey (1997) showed that people overwhelmingly want to reclaim and reassert the spiritual dimension in dying. Survey respondents said they wanted warm relationships with their providers, to be listened to, to have someone with whom to share their fears and concerns, to have someone with them when they are dying, to be able to pray and have others pray for them, and to have a chance to say goodbye to loved ones. When asked what would worry them, they said not being forgiven by God or others, or the prospect of continued emotional and spiritual suffering. When asked about what would bring them comfort, they said they wanted to believe that death is a normal part of the life cycle and that they would live on through their relationships, their accomplishments, or their good works. They also wanted to believe that they had done their best in their life and that they would be in the presence of a loving God or higher power. It is as important for health care providers and other caretakers to talk with patients about these issues as it is to address the medical side of care. Numerous surveys (e.g., Ehman, Ott, Short, Ciampa & Hansen-Flaschen, 1999; McCord, Gilchrist, Grossman, King, McCormick, et al., 2004) have shown that patients want their physicians to talk with them about their spiritual needs.

Studies also suggest that spirituality may be helpful to people as they cope with dying or loss. For example, patients with advanced cancer who derived comfort from their religious and spiritual beliefs were more satisfied with their lives, were happier, and reported less pain (Yates, Chalmers, St. James, Follansbee, & McKegney, 1981). Women with breast cancer said that their spiritual beliefs helped them cope with their illness and with facing death (Roberts, Brown, Elkins, & Larson, 1997). We have found that spirituality also affects a patient's will to live (Tsevat, J. et al., 2003).

How does spirituality work to help people cope with dying? One mechanism might be through hope. Spirituality and religion help people find hope in the midst of the despair that often occurs in the course of serious illness and dying. The nature of hope can change during the course of an illness: Early on, the person might hope for a cure; later, when a cure becomes unlikely, the person might hope for time to finish projects or travel, the ability to make peace with loved ones and with God, and a peaceful death. Spiritual beliefs help people find meaning in the midst of suffering, and religions help them see their suffering in a larger theological framework (Puchalski & O'Donnell, 2005).

Medical professionals are starting to recognize the inadequacies in the health care system in terms of care of the dying. The American College of

Physicians—American Society of Internal Medicine End-of-Life Care Consensus Panel concluded that physicians should extend their care of these patients by attentiveness to psychosocial, existential, and spiritual suffering (Lo, Quill, & Tulsky, 1999). The Joint Commission on Accreditation of Health Care Organizations (JCAHO) requires that spiritual care be available for patients in hospitals (JCAHO, 1996).

Interest in spirituality in medicine has grown exponentially among medical educators in the past decade. In 1993, only one medical school had a course in spirituality and medicine; now, over 70% of medical schools offer such courses. The key elements of these courses are listening to what is important to the patient, respecting patients' spiritual beliefs, and communicating effectively with patients about their spiritual beliefs and their preferences at the end of life.

In 1998, the Association of American Medical Colleges (AAMC), responding to concerns in the medical community that young doctors lacked humanitarian skills, undertook a major initiative: the Medical School Objectives Project. The project report notes that "Physicians must be compassionate and empathetic in caring for patients...they must act with integrity, honesty, respect for patients' privacy and respect for the dignity of patients as persons. In all of their interactions with patients, they must seek to understand the meaning of the patients' stories in the context of the patients' and family and cultural values" (AAMC, 1998, p. 2).

Physicians and health care professionals have an obligation to respond to and attempt to relieve the suffering of their patients. To this end, they should communicate with their patients about the patients' spirituality and how they are coping with suffering. Our systems of care should allow people to age gracefully and die in peace; to die the way they want to, including engaging in activities that bring peace to them, such as prayer, meditation, music, art, journaling, and sacred ritual.

SPIRITUAL ISSUES OF AGING AND DYING

At the end of life, spiritual issues come up for many people. Health care providers can gain insight into these issues from the dying person's spiritual history or from talking with the person about what he or she is experiencing emotionally and spiritually. Some of these issues are amenable to clinical intervention; however, unlike the use of certain medications for certain physical pain, standardized solutions do not exist for spiritual issues. Most of the work in dealing with these issues is done by the patients themselves, as part of their spiritual journey. Caregivers—professionals, family, and friends—can be present in a supportive and compassionate role. People may address the same issues many times; for example, there is no linear point at which one experiences hope and never again feels hopeless. Spiritual journeys are dynamic and fluid, and issues are revisited. However, over time there is usually some resolution. The following are some of the spiritual issues faced by chronically ill and dying patients:

- Lack of meaning and purpose in life
- Hopelessness
- Despair
- Fear of not being remembered
- Guilt, shame, and punishment
- Anger at God or others
- Feeling abandoned by God or others
- Feeling out of control
- Spiritual or existential suffering

Lack of Meaning and Purpose in Life

Patients may raise questions in the clinical setting that touch on this important theme. Why is this happening to me? Of what value is my life now? People may have found meaning and purpose in their work, their relationships, their avocations, and their attendance at church, temple, or mosque. Now they may no longer be able to work, pursue their hobbies, or attend their place of worship. Family and friends may have died or may not be very supportive. How can the patient find meaning in a world in which he or she no longer actively participates? How can patients continue to feel valued when the people and activities that made them feel valuable are no longer present or possible?

When people face their dying, they may realize what is most meaningful to them. That meaning is often derived from values, beliefs, practices, and experiences that have led them to an awareness of God/Divine/Holy/Transcendence and a sense of the ultimate value and purpose in life. In terms of Fowler's sixth stage, this sense of meaning may lead to a transference from reliance on others' beliefs and values to a stronger sense of one's own beliefs and values, and a move from dependence on self to dependence on a higher power. The universal values of love, justice, peace, and acceptance become prominent.

The goal in treatment is to help patients find that deeper meaning and feel the intrinsic value of themselves as human beings. Cognitive-oriented therapy can help, as well as referral to chaplains, pastoral counselors, and spiritual directors. (A spiritual director is a person who has been trained in spirituality, religion, and spiritual/faith development. They work with people on their spiritual or faith journeys. The focus of their work is on the relationship the person they are working with has with the transcendent God/Divine/Holy).

Health care professionals can ask questions such as these:

- What have been the important events in your life?

- What was the most important event in your life?

- What people have you loved?

- What is your relationship with a transcendent being or concept (God for religious patients; other spiritual or existential concepts for nonreligious patients)? Does this concept or relationship provide a sense of peace and meaning in your life?

Hopelessness

As people age and deal with infirmities or as they face their dying, loss of hope is common. Especially when they know that a cure is not possible, deep hopelessness may set in. But hope can be expressed in many ways. It may initially be for a cure, but if that is not possible, people may still find hope in finishing important projects, making peace with others, and having a peaceful death. This is where spirituality plays a vital role. The source of healing—the ability to become whole and hope-filled—is within each person. Everyone has the ability to heal, but people may need to be empowered and supported to find that inner resource.

Health care professionals can help by talking with patients about their past experiences with hope and helping them find new sources of hope. Helping patients create a dream list is one way to refocus their thinking in a more optimistic vein, even in the face of difficult situations. For religious people, religions talk about hope in the context of theological principles and relationship with God or a transcendent concept. For these people, referral to chaplains and pastoral counselors may be helpful.

Despair

When confronted with the possibility of dying, many people panic. Death is uncharted territory—a journey each person takes alone. It is normal to be frightened and filled with despair and a sense of not knowing where to turn. The most powerful intervention is listening to patients' fears, anxieties, and despair. It is important to be committed to being there for the patient for as long as it takes. The heavy load of despair is lightened for patients if they know that the physician and other health care professionals will be there to listen. People seek connection and unconditional love. Spiritual care is, at its essence, profound relationship-centered care. Offering altruistic love and compassion can help people move through despair. Other interventions might include chaplain referral and suggesting prayer, meditation, or other spiritual practices. Our society uses phrases like "giving up" or "losing the battle" to refer to dying, which in itself tends to promote despair. If we can help patients reframe the experience to see it as a natural phase of living, in which one accepts the process and gracefully allows it to happen, then letting go becomes the honorable way to face dying. It is not the loss of a battle but the successful accomplishment of a holy phase of living.

Fear of Not Being Remembered

One of the most common issues that people face as they age and die is the desire to be remembered (VandeCreek & Land Nye, 1994). People want to be remembered either through their work, the influence they've had, or their relationships. It is often helpful to ask patients how this might happen for them. A person might respond to the idea of telling his or her story into a tape recorder, or writing about his or her life. Some people find it helpful to make videos with messages for their loved ones. Others compose music, write poetry, or create visual art. Some people simply want to reconnect with family and friends in a special way. It is not uncommon to adjust therapy to enable people to accomplish their dreams and help them find ways to be remembered.

Guilt, Shame, and Punishment

Some people view their infirmities or their dying as a punishment or curse. This dynamic is important to uncover, as it can impede the treatment of symptoms; for example, some patients may refuse pain medication out of a belief that they deserve to die in pain. Listening for themes of guilt and a sense of being punished is important. One can ask about the patient's relationship with God. If God is punitive, the patient will not be able to go to God for help. People may be misinterpreting what their religion says about sin and punishment. A chaplain or pastoral counselor can help change the image of a punishing God.

Often, people's experience with their parents or others in their lives affects how they have come to understand God. These issues can be dealt with in therapy, but this takes time, so it is important to be supportive, accepting, and patient. Strong feelings about punishment often come from shame. As people talk about shame, they may come to a new awareness concerning events in their lives that led to the feeling of shame. They may be able to bring an adult perspective to these events, forgive themselves, and move on.

Anger at God or Others

Anger at God or others is a normal expression of the frustration of not being in control of one's life. In the Bible, Job calls out to God in despair over his plight. God listens to Job's complaints and anger, and never punishes him for these feelings. Instead, God points out that Job lacks the understanding to comprehend the reasons for his suffering. Eventually Job understands that the only solution to his suffering is complete trust that God will take care of him.

Let patients reveal their feelings, including anger. Bringing these deep emotions into the light may help the patient confront his or her sense of helplessness. But people need to move through this process themselves;

sometimes the anger is not resolved and the person dies angry. In her groundbreaking book *On Death and Dying*, Elizabeth Kubler-Ross noted that as long as the anger is a person's genuine expression of himself or herself, it does not need to be corrected. Each person has his or her own path to follow, and anger may be part of a patient's natural journey to death (Kubler-Ross, 1997).

Feeling Abandoned by God or Others

Dying is something one does alone, and a sense of abandonment is often seen in patients. Even Jesus felt abandoned by God ("Why have you forsaken me?"), so it is not surprising that patients may feel abandoned by God or by loved ones. As a spiritual experience, this can be considered the final purification of faith—having no proof, one still believes. But the sense of abandonment also may have roots in family life, and a lot of issues may come up from childhood. In response to the feeling of abandonment, a person may work through the despair and end up with a deeper belief or may conclude that the most important thing is to be at peace with God. If we offer patients comfort and our presence and support, they will feel less alone and more comfortable in the solitude of their dying. If the patient feels abandoned by God and loved ones, it is even more important to give that person the unconditional love he or she needs to feel supported. Come as a loving presence and help patients see love in God and others.

Feeling Out of Control

Aging and dying can provoke a deep sense of lack of control. One may have minimal control over the decisions that affect one: dressing, eating, bathing, and even bodily functions. Certainly, the ultimate lack of control comes in the moment of dying. We can help patients come to terms with these aspects of life. Certain spiritual belief systems see this process as detachment and a way to help people experience the greater spiritual virtues of love and dependence on nonmaterial aspects of life. While a patient may not be able to bathe himself, he can bask in the warmth of someone else's loving hands and have a profound sense of that love. It is very difficult to maintain dignity in the midst of some of the unattractive aspects of dying; thus, one of the most important clinical interventions is to help patients feel dignified and respected. Being a compassionate, loving presence with genuine respect for patients will help them.

Helping people find ways to control the things they can and be at peace with the things they cannot control can make a major difference in their lives. Religious/spiritual beliefs may help people find a sense of control; especially if they believe they are in God's care. Twelve-Step programs talk about turning things over to a higher power; "turning it over" can help people feel more in control of what seems like a disordered life (Anonymous, 1976).

Spiritual or Existential Suffering

Some people suffer deep existential or spiritual pain that may come from a sense of meaninglessness, hopelessness, despair, and unmet needs. It is important to talk with the patient to determine the source of the distress. But the pain may be coming from a profound spiritual crisis. St. John of the Cross, a 16th century mystic, wrote of the "dark night of the soul," when the pain is so intense that it may be unbearable (Collected Works of St. John of the Cross, 1991, pp. 402-403). This type of profound spiritual distress may be the way to enlightenment; in fact, some religions see such suffering as necessary for redemption. Religious tenets may help patients frame their suffering in a way that helps them deal with it. It is important for the health care professional to honor spiritual journeys, however difficult they may appear. To medicate these experiences as if they are merely physical pain, or experiences that can be "fixed" or avoided, may do the patient spiritual injustice.

Many aspects of dying are unknown and, thus, a mystery. Profound spiritual crises may well be in the realm of mystery. However, we can help patients by keeping them company and supporting them through these journeys. Listening to them, respecting their beliefs, and asking what might relieve the suffering are ways we can help the patient find healing. Prayer, music, nature, and art can all be used to help people tap into the spiritual stirring within.

LIFE FOR THE SPIRIT

How do patients move through the stages of dying in a spiritual way? By looking at the questions serious illness triggers and attempting to find answers to these questions for themselves. Most of the questions have no specific answers, and many lead to other questions. For example, "Why is this happening to me?" may lead to a life review and new insights that help people understand themselves or the Divine in a new way. "Who am I?" may be the impetus for a deeper search into self, with a resultant deeper understanding of self. Reconciliation and forgiveness may be the key elements in achieving inner peace and intimacy with God and others. Finally, confrontation with one's mortality may engender hope for living on, either eternally or through other people or one's accomplishments. I use an acronym—LIFE—to summarize the steps in this process:

LIFE for the Spirit®
Life review
Identity
Forgiveness/reconciliation
Eternity

A *life review* includes an analysis of one's past, in which people reflect on their relationships, accomplishments, and dreams, both lost and gained. Many issues come up for people during this review, such as failed or problematic relationships, perceived career failures, unaccomplished dreams, and regrets. People may become depressed or anxious during this time. Some experience guilt and anger. Some people are able to forgive; others hold a grudge and may isolate from others, especially loved ones. It is critical to address all dimensions of care. Depression may need to be treated with counseling and/or medication. A forgiveness intervention may be appropriate. Spiritual issues need to be identified and worked on with a chaplain or other health care provider. Ideally, people should be given all the resources they need to address these issues and achieve some resolution.

Identity refers to the questions people ask about who they are and what gives their life meaning. Often, as described in many of the patient stories, people find a deeper sense of who they are; usually, it is more congruous with their inner self than any definition they used in earlier parts of their lives. The realization that one may die or is dying affords one the opportunity to go deeper, to pause and reflect and, perhaps, to discover a new self.

Forgiveness plays an important role in each of our lives, on a personal as well as relational and societal levels. Forgiveness of ourselves can help us achieve an inner peace as well as peace with others and with God. Wrongdoing against others can result in guilt, self-recrimination, and self-loathing; perceived wrongdoing against us can create a distance or disconnect between self and others. Forgiveness is the first stage of self-love and acceptance. It is also the basic building block of loving relationships with others (Puchalski, 2002).

Eternity refers to the variety of beliefs people have about what happens after we die. Some people believe they will live on through others, such as family. Others have a sense that life continues through the actions we took while we were alive. Still others have religious concepts of a life after death, or reincarnation.

In addition to LIFE, several other tools can be used to discuss spiritual issues with patients; these include FICA (Puchalski & Romer, 2000) as described below, SPIRIT (Maugans, 1996), and HOPE (Anandarajah & Hight, 2001). A spiritual history can be taken as part of the patient's social history in the intake exam or annual physical or annual medical exam. The following are the goals of the spiritual history:

- Invite the patient to share spiritual and religious beliefs.

- Learn about the patient's beliefs and values.

- Assess for spiritual distress (sense of meaninglessness, hopelessness, etc.) and for spiritual resources (hope, sense of meaning and purpose, resiliency, spiritual community).

- Provide an opportunity for compassionate care through which the health care professional connects to the patient in a profound way.

- Empower the patient to find inner resources of healing and acceptance.

- Learn about the patient's spiritual and religious beliefs that might affect health care decision making.

FICA is a spiritual history tool I developed with several colleagues. It can be used in a time-efficient manner.

FICA: Taking a Spiritual History©

F = ***Faith and belief.*** "Do you consider yourself spiritual or religious?" or "Do you have spiritual beliefs that help you cope with stress?" If the patient says "No," the physician might ask, "What gives your life meaning?" Sometimes patients respond with answers such as family, career, or nature.

I = ***Importance.*** "What importance does faith or belief have in your life? Have your beliefs influenced how you take care of yourself in this illness? What role do your beliefs play in regaining your health?"

C = ***Community.*** "Are you part of a spiritual or religious community? Is this helpful to you; if so, how? Is there a group of people you really love or who are important to you?" Communities such as churches, temples, and mosques, or a group of like-minded friends can serve as a strong support system for some patients.

A = ***Address in care.*** "How would you like me, your health care provider, to address these issues in your health care?" Often it is not necessary to ask this question but simply to think about the spiritual issues that need to be addressed in the treatment plan, such as referral to chaplains, pastoral counselors, or spiritual directors; journaling; and music or art therapy. Sometimes the plan may include simply listening to and supporting the person in his or her journey.

CONCLUSION

Our culture needs to look at aging and dying very differently from the way it currently does. We need to see aging and dying as a natural part of life that can be meaningful and peaceful. People who are aging and dying should hold honored and special places in our society. Rather than spend so much energy avoiding aging and death, we can focus on our lives as spiritual journeys and concentrate on how we can age and die gracefully. We all need to live life now, knowing that one day we will die. By thinking about our mortality early in life, we will not be caught off guard and pressured by dilemmas and choices at the end of life. We can ask the deep spiritual questions long before we are on our deathbeds. This is where religious organizations can be particularly helpful. They can facilitate our discussions of dying and what that means to us. They can educate their members about the importance of preparing themselves for the choices, both spiritual and medical, that need to be made near the end of life. We can jointly help the dying person come to peace in life's last moments.

Our health care system needs to treat spirituality as essential to care—the spiritual experience is just as important as the physical experience of illness, aging, and dying. Fundamental to spiritual care is the relationship-centered care that all health care professionals provide. At the root of this care is the deep and profound respect we show each other and our patients. That respect transcends people's status or accomplishments. Imagine a health care system grounded in spiritual values of compassion and genuine respect for others. Such a health care system would provide the elements necessary for healing. ■

Christina M. Puchalski, MD, FACP, has pioneered the development of numerous educational programs for undergraduate, graduate, and postgraduate medical education in spirituality and medicine and spirituality and end-of-life care. Her spirituality curriculum at George Washington University was one of the first in the country and received the John Templeton Award for Spirituality and Medicine. Since 1996, she has directed a national award program for medical school curricula in spirituality and health. Dr. Puchalski is a practicing physician, board certified in internal medicine and palliative care. She is co-chair of a national education conference co-sponsored by the Association of American Medical Colleges and course co-director of Harvard Medical School and the Mind/Body Medical Institute's annual Spirituality & Healing in Medicine conference. Dr. Puchalski has recently published a new book on care for chronically ill and dying patients.

REFERENCES

Anonymous. (1976). *Alcoholics anonymous* (3rd ed.). New York: Alcoholics Anonymous World Services.

Anandarajah, G., & Hight, E. (2001). Spirituality and medical practice: Using the HOPE questions as a practical tool for spiritual assessment. *American Family Physician, 63*, 81-89.

Association of American Medical Colleges (AAMC). (1998). *Learning objectives for medical student education: Guidelines for medical schools* (Medical School Objectives Project report). Washington, D.C.: Author.

Brown, R. A. (1986). Reinhold Niebuhr: His theology in the 1980s. *Christian Century, 103*(6), 66-72.

Chandler, E. (1999). Spirituality. *Hospice Journal, 14*(3/4), 63-74.

Collected Works of St. John of the Cross. (1991). (K. Kavanaugh & O. Rodriquez, Trans.). Washington, DC: ICS Publications.

Ehman, J. W., Ott, B. B., Short, T. H., Ciampa, R. C., & Hansen-Flaschen, J. (1999). Do patients want their physicians to inquire about their spiritual or religious beliefs if they become gravely ill? *Archives of Internal Medicine, 159*, 1803-1806.

Fowler, J. W. (1981). *Stages of faith: The psychology of human development and the quest for meaning.* New York: Harper and Row.

Frankl, V. E. (1984). *Man's search for meaning.* New York: Simon and Schuster.

Gallup International Institute. (1997). *Spiritual beliefs and the dying process* (report on a national survey conducted for the Nathan Cummings Foundation and the Fetzer Institute). Philadelphia, PA: The Gallup International Institute.

Joint Commission on Accreditation of Health Care Organizations (JCAHO). (1996). *Implementation sections of the 1996 standards for hospitals.* Oakbrook Terrace, IL: JCAHO.

Kubler-Ross, E. (1997). *On death and dying* (1st Touchstone ed.). New York: Scribner Book Company.

Lo, B., Quill, T., & Tulsky, J. (1999). Discussing palliative care with patients. ACP-ASIM [American College of Physicians—American Society for Internal Medicine] End-of-Life Care Consensus Panel. *Annals of Internal Medicine, 130,* 744-749.

Maugans, T. A. (1996, January). The SPIRITual history. *Archives of Family Medicine, 3,* 11-16.

McCord, G., Gilchrist, V. J., Strossman, S. D., King, B. D., McCormick, K. E., Oprandi, A. M. (2004). Discussing spirituality with patients: A rational and ethical approach. *Annals of Family Medicine, 2*(4), 356-361.

Puchalski, C. M. (2002). Forgiveness: Spiritual and medical implications. *The Yale Journal for Humanities in Medicine, 17,* 1-6.

Puchalski, C. M., & O'Donnell, E. (2005). Religious and spiritual beliefs in end-of-life care: How major religions view death and dying. *Techniques in Regional Anesthesia and Pain Management, 9,* 114-121.

Puchalski, C. M., & Romer, A. L. (2000). Taking a spiritual history allows clinicians to understand patients more fully. *Journal of Palliative Medicine, 3,* 129-137.

Roberts, J. A., Brown, D., Elkins, T., & Larson, D. B. (1997). Factors influencing views of patients with gynecologic cancer about end-of-life decisions. *American Journal of Obstetrics and Gynecology, 176*(1), 166-172.

Tsevat, J., Puchalski, C. M., Sherman, S. N., Holmes, W. C., Feinberg, J., Leonard, A. C., Mrus, J. M., Mandell, K. L., Pargament, K.I., Justice, A. C., Fultz, S. L., Ellison, C. G., McCullough, M.E., Peterman, A. H. (2003). Spirituality and religion in patients with HIV/AIDS. *Journal of General Internal Medicine, 18* (Suppl. 1), 234-236.

VandeCreek, L., & Land Nye, C. (1994). Trying to live forever: Correlates to the belief in life after death. *Journal of Pastoral Care, 48*(3), 46-53.

Wald, F. S. (1986). In search of the spiritual component of hospice care. In F. S. Wald (Ed.), *In search of the spiritual component of hospice care* (pp. 25-33). New Haven, CT: Yale University Press.

Yates, J. W., Chalmers, B. J., St. James, P., Follansbee, M., & McKegney, F. P. (1981). Religion in patients with advanced cancer. *Medical and Pediatric Oncology, 9,* 121-128.

COMPLEMENTARY THERAPIES

When my father was no longer responding to curative treatment, his doctor suggested we call hospice. We did, and hospice has been successful in relieving much of his pain but my father's spirits are not good. His hospice suggested that we use other services the hospice provides—a social worker, chaplain, and a even massage and music therapist. I want to use everything available to help ease my father's pain, but I'm not sure about these other therapies, which I see as non-traditional. Will these other approaches really help?

■   ■   ■

One of the gifts of hospice is a holistic understanding and treatment of pain. Pain is not simply a physical sensation. Often psychological and spiritual factors contribute to pain. Complementary therapies can be very helpful in cases like your father's. Complementary therapies are used to help relieve stress and tension, to aid relaxation and to promote a sense of well being. Often, they are used in conjunction with medical treatment for patients. Some hospices make complementary therapies available to family members of the dying family member as well.

For example, if your father is anxious, fearful, or depressed, he could be more sensitive to physical pain. This can set up a destructive cycle: physical pain triggers anxiety that exacerbates pain; the pain inhibits rest and causes irritability; irritability drives others away and creates increased loneliness, anxiety, and depression. With less diversion, pain increases.

So spiritual, social, and psychological assessments are an important part of pain assessment. If spiritual or other concerns are troubling your father, speaking with a chaplain or a social worker may very well ease his mind, actually lessening his pain.

continued

Hospices have pioneered the use of complementary therapies such as art, music, or massage therapies. Other complementary therapies include hypnotheraphy, which uses hypnosis to reduce pain, nausea, anxiety, vomiting, and depression. "Energy work" is a term used to describe a variety of ancient and modern approaches to the theory that the body is composed of energy fields. Acupuncture, Reiki, and Shiatsu, as well as therapeutic touch can be used in energy work.

These therapies are called "complementary" therapies because they are used along with (rather than instead of) pharmaceutical approaches to pain control. These therapeautic services are also commonly known as "bodywork."

Some, such as massage therapy, may have a direct role in pain management—easing sore or tight muscles and stimulating circulation. Massage therapy transmits a sense of caring to the patient, which can help to promote a sense of physical and emotional well being. Others, such as music therapy, may have a more indirect yet important role in easing pain, offering effective diversion. You or your father can initiate these therapies if desired— increasing a sense of personal control at this difficult time.

Often, we hear about the mind-body connection. Music, colors, a much-loved pet, and even aromas can have physiological effects decreasing stress and even lower physical signs of stress such as pulse rate or blood pressure. Remember, together these approaches do more than simply treat the pain— they treat the person. You have made a good choice by selecting hospice. Hospice has already shown you how effective it can be in making your father comfortable. Carefully consider all the options it can offer.

■ CHAPTER 4 ■

Social, Cultural, Spiritual, and Psychological Barriers to Pain Management

By Kenneth J. Doka

INTRODUCTION

In 1986, a statement from the World Health Organization (WHO) asserted, "Nothing would have a greater impact on improving cancer pain treatment than implementing current knowledge" (Herr, 2004). Sadly, 20 years later, that statement is no less true.

There is a powerful paradox in pain control. In the past 30 years, there has been extensive and worldwide growth in hospice and effective end-of-life palliative care. Pharmaceutical and other pain management strategies have been developed so that few people need experience extensive pain at the end of life. Yet, the reality is that many people die in pain every day (Bernabei et al., 1998).

How do we explain this paradox, especially in countries such as the United States, which would seem to have all the resources needed to provide good palliative care? The fact is that while the technology for pain control is there, there are many complex and interrelated barriers to effective pain management at the end of life. These barriers include social, spiritual, cultural, legal, regulatory, and educational obstacles to pain control. The barriers affect and impede not only physicians and other health care workers but also patients and their families.

A cultural gap exists in pain management: We know far more about the control of pain than we have effectively been able to incorporate into regular medical practice. This chapter explores that gap, identifying six types of barriers to effective pain control. The hope is that by identifying these obstacles we can overcome them and fully realize the vision of the late Dame Cicely Saunders, the founder of the modern hospice movement, who believed that people need not die in pain.

BARRIERS TO PAIN MANAGEMENT

Social Barriers

Since the early years of the 20th century, the government of the United States has actively sought to control the illegal use of certain drugs, such as opioids. This campaign has left the general population with a deep-seated negative impression of opium and opioid drugs. The use of such drugs carries a strong social stigma and opprobrium that leaves even those who need relief from constant terminal pain reluctant to turn to such pharmaceutical remedies. In an era when we are urged to "just say no," it is often difficult to say "yes" to opioids, even when there is a legitimate purpose for using them. In short, the general social climate looks at the use of drugs as a mark of weakness of character. The result is that even people in terminal pain (and their families) would rather tolerate pain than use medications that carry such a stigma.

The so-called "war on drugs" has not left the medical profession unscathed: Physicians may share the negative outlook. It is not unusual for physicians and other care providers to suspect that a patient who claims to be in pain even after being treated for an underlying condition may be a potential or active drug abuser (Hill, 1993). This attitude may persist even though the experience of pain is quite subjective and tolerance of pain medication varies among individuals.

Beyond the general social climate, physicians worry about the regulatory and legal implications of prescribing opioids. These drugs are highly regulated and controlled, and physicians know that the heavy use of opioids can call attention to one's practice. While this is more of an issue in chronic than in terminal care (especially hospice care), it still has a chilling effect. The restrictive regulatory and legal climate has generated calls to increase the availability of drugs, including opioids, to manage pain (Dilcher, 2004). Even the National Association of Attorneys General has recognized the need to assess the extent to which federal and state policies regulating controlled substances can inhibit pain management.

An additional social factor creates a barrier to pain management: income. It is well established that income generally affects access to all aspects of health care, including hospice and palliative care (Boyd & Clayton, 2002). Lower income persons are less likely to use hospice services and more likely to report pain at every level of care.

There are many reasons for this discrepancy. Lower income persons generally have fewer available health care alternatives. They may not know about medical alternatives such as hospice or about their right to receive these services. Lack of a primary care physician and dependence on clinics and emergency rooms may make it more difficult to offer and coordinate such services (Green, Baker, & Nday-Brumblay, 2004).

Other implications of social class and income may be subtler. For example, there is likely to be a significant social and educational disparity between physicians and lower income clients that may impair communication. Lower income clients may be afraid to assert themselves, unable to advocate when interacting with physicians, and more likely to respond to the physician's sense of authority. On their part, physicians may suspect that a lower income patient who constantly complains of pain and seeks opioids may, in fact, be a potential abuser.

Cultural Barriers

Another set of barriers to pain control is cultural. Since the 1965 Immigration Act, American society has become increasingly ethnically and culturally diverse, with increasing immigration from Asia, Africa, and South America. Cultural diversity can affect pain management in a number of ways.

There is some evidence that the very experience of pain may differ among cultures. Early research by Zborowski (1952) suggested that pain thresholds themselves might differ among cultural groups.

Beyond possible differences in pain thresholds, culture can create barriers in two ways. First, it may be difficult to effectively assess pain in persons of another culture. Pain is a highly subjective and individual experience, and it is never easy to assess another's experience of pain. The difficulty of assessing pain can become infinitely more pronounced when communicating across cultures. In certain cultures, pain is met with stoicism, so a lack of verbal or behavioral expressions of pain may not mean that the pain does not exist. In other cases, persons of different cultures, especially when English is not the first language, may not fully adhere to pharmaceutical treatments because they do not fully understand the instructions (Juarez, Ferrell, & Borneman, 1998).

Second, culture may influence adherence to pain management regimens. Persons from different cultures may have their own beliefs about the significance of pain, symptoms, treatment, and even the very meaning of disease. For example, Fadiman (1997) describes the cultural clash that occurred when American physicians sought to treat a Hmong child suffering from epilepsy. Her family was at first confused and nonadhering, because the medications prescribed seemed to make the child ill. More important, they were ambivalent about the treatment. In Hmong culture, epilepsy is considered a deeply spiritual experience; the epileptic is a highly honored, chosen conduit to the spiritual world. This story illustrates the fact that, to treat a person effectively, health care providers must be sensitive to the individual's cultural experience of illness.

This is true in pain management as well. Cultures may have their own beliefs about the importance and meaning of pain and their own folk remedies. The sensitive health care provider tries to understand these perspectives and, when possible, use them as adjuncts to treatment.

Again, physicians need to be aware of their own biases when they approach members of different cultures. Cultural differences can color assessments of the veracity and validity of the patient's pain complaints.

All of these social and cultural factors can interact. For example, Anderson et al. (2000) found in their study of economically disadvantaged African-American and Hispanic cancer patients that both groups were undertreated for pain by their physicians, and that undertreatment was most pronounced for female patients.

Spiritual Barriers

Pain and suffering have always been part of the human condition, and every faith and form of spirituality has addressed the question of why humans experience pain and suffering. The answers have varied. To some, suffering and pain are experiences that tie an individual to the whole of humanity; so to deny pain is to deny being human. As Moller writes:

> The normative medical response to pain is to demand more drugs, doctors and hospitals…. If humanity is deprived of the capacity to suffer, then it embarks on a path which narrows the experience of being human (1986, p. 129).

To others, pain is a mystical experience, one that brings the individual into a deeper connection with God. Still others see pain and suffering as retribution for acts committed in this or previous lives. To these believers, to deny pain is to fail to fulfill the tasks inherent in life and, thus, be doomed to repeat them in some future life or suffer in an afterlife. Aries (1981) reminds us that in the Middle Ages sudden death was most feared, as it deprived the individual of an opportunity to repent for his or her sins. Severe pain had value: Not only did the suffering motivate the individual to become right with God; it also lessened the time he or she would have to spend in Purgatory (where one was purged of sin as one awaited acceptance into Heaven).

In some belief systems with dual or multiple deities, pain might be attributed to the more malign spirit. In other systems, pain may be considered a warning from God or a path to new understanding or insight. Even many people with a nontheistic belief system see pain in the latter light. Fertziger (1986) makes no direct theistic reference as he asserts that pain at the end of life is the crucial link between death and growth. This widely held belief (an instrumental view of pain) emphasizes that pain is an essential instrument of growth. Without pain, there can be no change. Consider how pervasive this view is: It can be found all the way from Marxist theory, which holds that the suffering of the masses is essential for revolution, to the signs in a gym that proclaim "No pain, no gain."

Other spiritual belief systems affirm that pain is simply "fate," over which humans have little, if any, control. And some people believe that pain is simply a mystery—there is no answer to why we experience pain and suffering; we just do.

The point is that every individual—and, for that matter, every health care provider—has spiritual beliefs about the nature of pain and suffering. In many cases, these beliefs may include a perceived spiritual benefit to experiencing pain or suffering. It is essential to understand and assess these beliefs to provide effective pain management, as they may impede the delivery of pain relief.

Personal and Familial Barriers

While spiritual beliefs may interfere with effective pain management, other beliefs, knowledge, and attitudes held by the patient or by family caregivers also may inhibit pain control. Pain is subjective, and the only way it can be treated is if it is appropriately assessed. Thus, pain may not be effectively treated if conscious and aware patients either do not report or minimize their experience of pain.

There may be many reasons why patients do that. They may have fears about pain control. They may worry that pain medications will cloud their judgment, reduce their independence, or limit their level of consciousness. An Australian study, for example, found that older patients strongly wanted their physicians to explain options about pain management and actively involve them in developing regimens to control pain (Lansbury, 2000).

Patients also may be reluctant to admit to pain. They may believe that a good patient accepts discomfort and does not complain or that, in any case, effective management of the pain may not be available. They may harbor, even at the end of life, fears of addiction. There may be a social class or generational factor here as well: Patients who were less educated, reported lower income, or were older were more likely to hold these beliefs (Ward et al., 1993).

Other fears may need to be addressed. Patients may fear that the drugs will cause opioid toxicity; that is, they may fear the implications of regularly taking drugs that are often portrayed as dangerous. The multiple warning labels placed on such drugs, designed to discourage inappropriate use, may feed these fears (Bressler, Geraci, & Schatz, 1991). Patients may worry about tolerance, fearing that they will need to increase the dosage to levels that will be incapacitating. They may be fearful of procedures (unsure of dosages or fearful of injections) or worried about the implications of drug use. In short, many patient-related barriers may interfere with pain management (Dawson et al., 2005).

In addition to fears and lack of knowledge, patient attitudes must be considered. Patients may believe that it is a mark of courage and tenacity to die without medication. In Harper Lee's classic novel *To Kill a Mockingbird* (1960), there is a rather unpleasant character named Mrs. Dubose. At one point in the book, Jem Finch, the teenage son of the central character, has to read to this dying woman. To Jem, the experience becomes increasingly strange. Mrs. Dubose always begins by taunting and berating him, then falls into a strange silence. Later, Jem learns that, as she died, the old woman was attempting to break her illness-related addiction to morphine. Her decision to die in pain is cast as a great act of personal courage; a lesson in bravery for Jem and his sister Scout.

Some patients may be said to have the "Dubose syndrome"—a desire to die without medication, even if this decision results in a painful death. While this may be a legitimate choice by a patient with the capacity to make such a decision, it should always be assessed and discussed.

These fears, attitudes, and misinformation may exist not only in patients but in their family caregivers as well (Letizia, Creech, Norton, Shanahan & Hedges, 2004). In fact, the importance of caregiver beliefs and attitudes is magnified at the end of life, when they may be the primary administrators of pain medication and, in some cases, the primary source of information on the patient's pain.

Physician and Health Care Provider Barriers

But the major barriers to pain management rest with physicians and health care providers rather than with patients and their families. Dawson et al. (2005) found that while patients' beliefs were a factor in the effective management of pain, it was the health care providers' pain management behaviors that were most predictive of pain relief. Even with resistant patients, physicians and other health care providers could generally prevail. The paradox of pain management is most evident here: The tremendous increase in knowledge and resources to control pain has not effectively translated into medical practice (Weinstein et al., 2000).

This situation is partly owing to bias or, as Weinstein et al. term it, "opiophobia"—prejudice against the use of opioid analgesics. Beyond this bias regarding the use of opioid analgesics, physicians also may hold negative views regarding patients who constantly complain of pain (Weinstein et al., 2000). Often, too, they perceive that high dosages of opioid analgesics will attract unwelcome regulatory scrutiny of their practices (Hill, 1993).

It is not just bias, though; education is also a factor. The new Joint Commission on Accreditation of Healthcare Organizations (JCAHO) standards emphasize pain management, but many physicians and other health care providers were educated at a time when pain management and palliative care were not emphasized. Many providers lack skill in pain assessment or knowledge of the need to individualize the treatment of pain on the basis of the patient's profile. Many professionals may not understand appropriate analgesic regimens or the routing of dosing. Physicians and other health care providers lack information on standards and procedures for treating pain (Hill, 1993; Tarzian & Hoffmann, 2005; Weinstein et al., 2000). Some health care providers are uncomfortable administrating pain medication, fearing that they might overdose a patient (Tarzian & Hoffmann, 2005). Moreover, physicians and other health care providers may be confused and may find it difficult to differentiate among addiction, physical dependence, and tolerance (Weinstein et al., 2000). These factors further complicate the assessment and treatment of pain.

This kind of confusion, especially at the end of life, has led to perceived ethical dilemmas. Health care providers often struggle with such ethical concerns as euthanasia, assisted suicide, and terminal sedation; they are unsure of where moral boundaries could be drawn and confused about how their attempts to manage pain might be perceived (Ferrell et al., 2001).

Structural Barriers

The current structure of medical practice militates against effective pain management. Medical care, especially in the United States and other industrialized nations, is highly specialized. Dying persons, especially older persons, may have multiple chronic conditions for which they are seeing various specialists. Even within the treatment of one illness, patients may see multiple specialists. Furthermore, a patient may be treated in different settings—home, hospital, and nursing home—further limiting the continuity of care. The result is often a fragmentation of care. No one physician holds primary responsibility for the patient and his or her pain. Outside of hospice, multidisciplinary teams to manage pain are rare (Gaijchen, Blum, & Calder, 1995).

This fragmentation of care limits the communication between physicians and patients. Patients may not know their specialists very well. Even more critically, the physician may not know the patient, which further complicates the assessment of pain (Redmond, 1997). Fragmentation also can inhibit appropriate referrals to hospice, the institution most skilled in symptom control and pain management (Tarzian & Hoffmann, 2005).

There may be other structural difficulties as well. Pain may not be consistently kept track of (Redmond, 1997). Because opioids are so highly regulated, health care organizations may create additional procedures to document their prescription and administration. Such procedures may create a lack of flexibility and increase the time and work needed to administer pain medications, further impeding pain management (Carr, 1997; Redmond, 1997). These problems are exacerbated in facilities that suffer from ineffective or inconsistent leadership or poor working relationships among health care staff (Brockopp et al., 1998).

EASING THE PAIN: SUGGESTIONS FOR PRACTICE

Advances have been made in easing the pain of persons at the end of life. The development and growth of hospice over the past 30 years is a substantial accomplishment. Hospice has not only brought a vision to the public of living comfortably to the end of life; it has spawned both pharmaceutical and nonpharmaceutical strategies for alleviating pain and has modeled interdisciplinary and holistic care to treat pain. In fact, the growth of the hospice movement has generated a greater interest in palliative care.

There have been other advances as well. The WHO has made cancer pain relief one of its top priorities for research, education, and advocacy (McCaffery, 1992). The new JCAHO standards emphasize to hospitals and health care providers the primary importance of pain management. The efforts of the National Association of Attorneys General have called attention to the ways that regulatory practices and policies may inhibit the effective management of pain, possibly leading to changes in the overall regulatory climate that influences pain management.

Yet, much remains to do. Continued research is a major priority. That research should not only seek to develop new pharmaceutical methods of pain management but should also assess nonpharmaceutical and complementary approaches to pain control, the advantages and drawbacks of various routes of administration of pain medication, and the effectiveness of various strategies of pain management. For example, the notion of "pain ladders," in which one moves from one level to another, has been challenged with the suggestion that it may be necessary to "skip steps" after assessment to allow more timely and effective pain management. Obviously, research will be necessary to establish the claims of these different approaches to pain control. Pain research also should clearly evaluate pain management strategies and the effectiveness of medications on underserved populations such as older persons, women, and children. Psychosocial research is also needed. Training for health care providers in pain management, techniques for consumer education, and approaches to improving communication among health care providers, family caregivers, and patients all need to be developed and evaluated.

Research alone, though, is not enough. Pain management must be infused into the education of physicians, nurses, and other health care providers. Such training should include knowledge of the varied pharmaceutical and nonpharmaceutical approaches to pain management and the strategies to administer drugs. It should also strengthen the skills that enable physicians, nurses, and other health care providers to assess pain in patients. Skills training can range from a simple reminder that rephrasing a question from "Are you in pain?" to "Are you comfortable?" can yield more information to training in sophisticated approaches to assess and manage pain in populations such as persons with developmental disabilities or dementia. Physicians can be taught to include patients and families in an experimental ethos. Patients and families may be willing to try strategies that are clearly explained as trials, especially if they know that they will have a role in evaluating whether or not these medications will be continued. Training also should allow health professionals to confront their own biases that might affect pain management, including a reluctance to use opioid analgesics or discomfort with patients from other cultures or social classes.

Training of health professionals should include tools to help them approach patients and their families. Patients and families share responsibility for pain control; in fact, patient self-reports are the most important tools in pain assessment. When the patient is incapacitated, the observations of family caregivers are essential. The fears and concerns of patients and families may offer considerable barriers to effective pain management. Physicians, nurses, and other health professionals need training and supervision in communicating with the patients and their families and involving them in pain management.

Training is needed at all levels. Often, it is the home health aide or the nursing assistant who has the closest relationship with the patient and, thus, is the most suitable person to assess pain. Often, it is the aide who administers and monitors pain medication. The overall process of pain management will work best if these medical personnel are well-trained and valued.

Patient and family education is essential. Patients and family caregivers may need to be educated in ways to assess pain and administer medications. They may need to learn to be pain advocates for themselves or a family member. This process works best when patients and families have adequate training and are respected by health professionals.

But pain management is not just about individuals; systems will need to change as well. Pain management is the responsibility of everyone on the health care team. Many dying patients have multiple diagnoses and chronic conditions, so pain must be managed across medical disciplines and specialties. Unfortunately, especially in hospitals and nursing homes, systems may not facilitate or even allow such cross-communication. An emphasis on education would encourage communication across disciplines and specialties.

Hospitals, and sometimes nursing homes, often have one element that can take a more active role in pain management: the ethics committee. Ethics committees can help in three ways. First, they can encourage consultation among health professionals on pain management issues, even sponsoring grand rounds on the topic. Pain management and ethical concerns intersect at the end of life, especially in areas such as terminal sedation or fears (often needless) about addiction or euthanasia. Ethics committees can help health professionals grapple with their concerns and questions.

Second, ethics committees can be proactive. The very fact that a dying patient is experiencing significant pain may raise ethical issues. Ethics committees can examine the situation and offer a forum to educate health professionals, family caregivers, and patients.

Third, ethics committees should review each death to determine whether appropriate palliative care and timely referral to hospice services were offered. Such a practice would be an ongoing reminder to health care providers that no patient should die in needless, treatable pain.

CONCLUSION

Pain management is an emerging frontier in medicine and end-of-life care. There is no reason that a person should die in unnecessary pain. Such a death not only affects the dying person; it exacerbates the grief of survivors and creates increased anxiety about their own future deaths. The cycle of suffering extends beyond the patient.

Numerous barriers exist to effective pain management, but there are hopeful signs. Hospice has demonstrated both a technology and a practical approach consistent with its vision that people can live in relative comfort until they die. The hospice approach is spreading to other health care facilities, such as hospitals and nursing homes. That is the good news. The hope is that more and more people will benefit. ◾

Kenneth J. Doka, PhD, is a professor of gerontology at the Graduate School of the College of New Rochelle and senior consultant to the Hospice Foundation of America. A prolific author, Dr. Doka has written or edited 19 books and more than 60 articles and book chapters. He is the editor of Omega *and* Journeys: A Newsletter to Help in Bereavement.

Dr. Doka was elected president of the Association for Death Education and Counseling in 1993. In 1995, he was elected to the board of directors of the International Work Group on Dying, Death and Bereavement; he chaired the work group from 1997 through 1999. In 1994, he received the award for Outstanding Contributions in the Field of Death Education from the Association for Death Education and Counseling. Dr. Doka is an ordained Lutheran minister.

REFERENCES

Anderson, K., Mendoza, F., Valero, V., Richman, S., Russell, C., Hurley, J., et al. (2000). Minority cancer patients and their providers: Pain management attitudes and practice. *Cancer, 88*, 1929-1938.

Aries, P. (1981). *The hour of our death*. New York: Knopf.

Bernabei, R., Gambassi, G., Lapane, K., Landi, F., Gatsonis, C., Dunlop, R., et al. for the SAGE Study Group. (1998). Management of pain in elderly patients with cancer. *Journal of the American Medical Association, 279*, 1877-1892.

Boyd, M., & Clayton, L. (2002). *An American health dilemma: Race, medicine and health care in the United States, 1900-2000*. New York: Routledge.

Bressler, L., Geraci, M., & Schatz, B. (1991). Misperceptions and inadequate pain management in cancer patients. DICP. *Annals of Pharmacology, 25*, 1225-1230.

Brockopp, D., Brockopp, G., Warden, S., Wilson, J., Carpenter, J., & Vandeveer, B. (1998). Barriers to change: A pain management project. *International Journal of Nursing Studies, 35*, 226-232.

Carr, E. (1997). Structural barriers to pain control. *Nursing Times, 93*(41), 50-51.

Dawson, R., Sellers, D., Spross, J., Jablonski, E., Hoyer, D., & Solomon, M. (2005). Do patients' beliefs act as barriers to effective pain management behaviors and outcomes inpatients with cancer-related or non-cancer-related pain? *Oncology Nursing Forum, 32*(2), 363-374.

Dilcher, A. (2004). Damned if they do, damned if they don't: The need for comprehensive public policy to address the inadequate management of pain. *Annals of Health Law, 13*, 81-144.

Fadiman, A. (1997). *The spirit catches you and you fall down: A Hmong child, her American doctors and the collision of two cultures*. New York: Farrar, Straus and Giraux.

Ferrell, B., Novy, D., Sullivan, M., Banja, J., DuBois, M., Gitlin, M., et al. (2001). Ethical dilemmas in pain management. *Journal of Pain, 2,*171-180.

Fertziger, A. (1986). Death and growth: The problem of pain. In R. DeBellis, E. Marcus, C. Smith Torres, V. Barrett, & M. Siegel (Eds.), *Suffering: Psychological and social aspects in loss, grief, and care* (pp. 141-150). New York: Haworth Press.

Gaijchen, M., Blum, D., & Calder, K. (1995). Cancer pain management and the role of social work: Barriers and interventions. *Health and Social Work, 20,* 200-206.

Green, C., Baker, T., & Nday-Brumblay, S. (2004). Patient attitudes regarding healthcare utilization and referral: A descriptive comparison in African and Caucasian Americans with chronic pain. *Journal of the National Medical Association, 96*(1), 31-42.

Herr, K. (June 2004). *Geriatric pain: Assessment and treatment strategies.* Presentation to the 16th Annual Meeting of the American Alliance of Cancer Pain Initiatives, St. Louis, MO.

Hill, C., Jr. (1993). The barriers to adequate pain management with opioid analgesics. *Seminars in Oncology, 20* (Suppl. 1), 1-5.

Juarez, G., Ferrell, B., & Borneman, T. (1998). The influence of culture on cancer pain management in Hispanic patients. *Cancer Practice, 6*(5), 282-289.

Lansbury, G. (2000). Chronic pain management: A qualitative study of elderly people's preferred coping strategies and barriers to treatment. *Disability and Rehabilitation, 22,* 2-14.

Lee, H. (1960) *To kill a mockingbird.* New York: J.B. Lippincott.

Letizia, M., Creech, S., Norton, E., Shanahan, M., & Hedges, L. (2004). Barriers to caregiver administration of pain medication in hospice care. *Journal of Pain and Symptom Management, 27,* 114-124.

McCaffery, M. (1992). Pain control: Barriers to the use of available information. *Cancer, 70* (Suppl. 5), 1438-1449.

Moller, D. W. (1986).On the value of suffering in the shadow of death. In R. DeBellis, E. Marcus, C. Smith Torres, V. Barrett, & M. Siegel (Eds.), *Suffering: Psychological and social aspects in loss, grief, and care* (pp. 127-136). New York: Haworth Press.

Redmond, K. (1997). Organizational barriers in opioid use. *Supportive Care in Cancer, 5,* 451-456.

Tarzian, A., & Hoffmann, D. (2005). Barriers to managing pain in the nursing home: Findings from a statewide survey. *Journal of the American Medical Directors Association, 6* (Suppl. 3), S13-S19.

Ward, S., Goldberg, N., Miller-McCauley, V., Mueller, C., Nolan, A., Pawlik-Plank, D., et al. (1993). Patient-related barriers to management of cancer pain. *Pain, 52,* 319-324.

Weinstein, S., Laux, L., Thornby, J., Lorimor, R., Hill, C. Jr., Thorpe, D., et al. (2000). Physicians' attitudes toward pain and the use of opioid analgesics: Results of a survey from the Texas Cancer Pain Initiative. *Southern Medical Journal, 93,* 479-487.

Zborowski, M. (1952). Cultural components in responses to pain. *Journal of Social Issues, 8,* 16-30.

SECTION II

The Assessment and Management of Pain

This is the largest section in the book and, in a sense, the heart of the volume.

Pain management begins with assessment. John Mulder, MD, provides an overview of effective approaches to assessing pain.

In Chapter 6, Keela Herr, PhD, and Sheila Decker, PhD, describe ways health practitioners can assess pain in a patient with cognitive impairment. Herr and Decker explore indirect methods of pain assessment, such as the use of family and other surrogate reports, direct observation of possible pain indicators, changes in activities, and analgesic trials. Their work challenges the myth that people with cognitive impairments may not experience severe pain. As the "Beyond Theory" inquiry at the end of the chapter shows, assessment can be very difficult in cases where the patient cannot report his or her condition. Observations of family members and caregivers can be a useful adjunct to the medical assessment process.

The myth surrounding the experience of pain has affected other populations, too, such as infants: In the past, there was a general belief that the infant's nervous system was too underdeveloped to experience severe pain. Rebecca Selove, a clinical psychologist; Dianne Cochran, a nurse; and Ira Todd Cohen, a physician, team up to write a chapter on assessing and managing pain in children and adolescents. The authors address the unique challenges inherent in pain assessment in these populations and describe sound practices for managing children's pain.

In the next chapter, Arthur G. Lipman, PharmD, considers pharmaceutical approaches to pain management at the end of life. This chapter is a primer on pain management, as Lipman not only reviews pharmaceutical strategies and principles for relieving pain but also summarizes some of the current debates about how best to approach pain at the end of life.

Janet L. Abrahm, MD, uses a case study approach to illustrate approaches, advances and pitfalls in pain management as part of end-of-life care. Abrahm describes how pharmaceutical and nonpharmaceutical strategies can work together for effective pain management. Abrahm's chapter illustrates a critical point. Effective pain control requires an experimental orientation—a willingness to continue to reassess and to modify treatment plans when the patient's needs change and until effective pain control is achieved.

While advocating strongly for the use of an array of strategies to treat pain, Abrahm is sensitive to the policy implications: Reimbursement may be difficult to secure for some complementary services.

Abrahm's ideas are expanded in the next two chapters. Donna Kalauokalani, MD, provides a survey of complementary therapies that can be used to supplement pharmaceutical strategies. While the data are limited, evidence exists of the usefulness of many of these approaches. At the very least, such approaches may relieve stress and stress-related symptoms that might exacerbate pain. Such strategies may improve a sense of therapeutic alliance between the patient and health teams as such approaches often are compatible with the patient's cultural beliefs and practices. Additionally, these strategies can provide diversion and give patients and family members a sense of control at a very chaotic time.

While Kalauokalani's chapter does not exclusively focus on the end of life, many of the therapies she addresses have been effectively used by hospice at the end of life. There are, however, important differences. For hospice, for example, nutrition is far more than an adjunct to therapy—it is a core service. Registered dieticians are a critical part of the hospice team in at least two ways. First, registered dieticians fully participate in the development of care plans, making recommendations about feeding, hydration, and nutrition. They facilitate pain management by offering nutritional counseling that may reduce constipation and other side effects of medication or other side effects of treatment. Second, when the goal becomes palliative, dieticians serve as advocates, urging families to provide favorite foods and meals, thereby enhancing comfort at the end of life.

Samira K. Beckwith, LCSW, CEO, and president of the Hope Hospice of Southwest Florida, concludes this section with an overview of the hospice approach to pain control. Beckwith provides an excellent description of a hospice team at work—each member, from physician to volunteer, contributing unique talents and abilities to the assessment, management, and relief of pain. Beckwith's chapter echoes a theme that runs throughout this section of the book: Pain is a multifaceted experience involving not only physical sensations but also psychological, spiritual, social, financial, cultural, and familial factors. Physical pain cannot be assessed or treated in isolation.

Beckwith reiterates another critical point as well: The pain that a patient experiences (or that the family perceives that the patient experiences) affects the entire family. Family members suffer along with the patient; thus, pain management is a family issue. Moreover, this suffering may continue long after the patient's death, as families struggle with grief, with guilt about their inability to relieve their loved one's pain, and with existential questions of why their relative suffered. The effective management of pain includes alleviating the psychological and spiritual pain of survivors, and facilitating the grieving process. The bereavement care that hospice provides is a very important part of the total picture of end-of-life pain management. ■

■ CHAPTER 5 ■

Comprehensive Pain Assessment

John Mulder

INTRODUCTION

Pain pervades the human spirit. It invades the body and cripples the psyche. No one can avoid the reality, the presence, or the specter of pain. One of the conundrums of the practice of medicine is that in the context of the ubiquitous nature of pain, and despite the abundance of effective modalities of treatment available for the relief of pain, too many people continue to suffer. Pain remains undertreated by many practitioners.

A number of explanations are offered for the gap between pain and relief, among them the following: inadequate knowledge on the part of practitioners who treat those in pain, fear of regulatory reprisal for prescribing opioids for pain control, patients' reluctance to admit they are in pain and submit to recommended protocols, and discomfort among staff who are responsible for administering opioids and other pain-relieving therapies. However, the most important factor in the process of achieving appropriate control of pain is assessment. Assessment allows for full understanding of the nature, meaning, source, and character of pain; without that understanding, efforts to relieve suffering will always fall short. While pain is commonly assigned to a category (acute, chronic, cancer, postoperative) that allows for the development of optimal treatment strategies, the components of a comprehensive assessment are common to all categories. This chapter will describe the essential aspects of a competent pain assessment.

WHAT IS PAIN?

Margo McCaffery's well-known description of pain—"Pain is whatever the experiencing person says it is, existing whenever he/she says it does" (McCaffery, 1968, p. 95)—underscores a fundamental principle of pain assessment: Believe the patient. Pain is not a diagnosis but rather a symptom, and the person who is experiencing pain has the right to define it in the manner that describes it for him or her. Because of their training, clinicians tend to feel more comfortable with objective measurements in assessing patients (e.g., a laboratory value, a radiological result, a physical finding on exam, an aberrant vital sign). A rapid pulse rate and elevated blood pressure might be present in an acute pain episode, but there is no objective finding or test that can confirm or refute the presence of pain. While malingering is seen in the rare patient and drug-seeking behaviors require vigilance on the part of practitioners, the vast majority of patients who complain of pain do, in fact, experience pain.

HISTORY AND PHYSICAL EXAMINATION

The medical history is unequivocally the most important factor in a comprehensive pain assessment. It is accomplished in the context of a general medical evaluation, including current and past health or illness, surgeries, current medications, and allergies. It must include the following components:

- The **chronology of the pain** must be established: When did it first appear? What triggered it? When it is present, how long does it last? When does it occur—during the day or night? Is it constant or intermittent, frequent or occasional?

- The **character of the pain** must be defined:
    - —*Location:* Where is the pain? Where does it appear to start, and where does it radiate? Is there a referred component? Is it deep or superficial?
    - —*Quality:* How does the person describe the pain (aching, gnawing, stabbing, sharp, dull, etc.)?
    - —*Intensity:* How severe is the pain? (See discussion of pain below.)
    - —*Provocative or relieving factors:* What makes the pain worse? What relieves it? What quantities and types of medication has the person taken? How effective (or ineffective) have they been?

- The **impact on the patient's activities and lifestyle** must be assessed: How does the pain affect mood, sleep and eating habits, activities of daily living, chores or work, and social activities? What is the impact on marriage, family, friendships, and other relationships?

It is important to select a pain rating scale that can be used to provide baseline information about a patient's pain and then also used to monitor symptom progression, improvement, and response to therapy. The same scale should be used with a patient throughout the pain management process to enhance the consistency and reliability of the assessment. Tools should be selected that can be used across the spectra of race, age, culture, and emotional or intellectual status.

The most common scale used by practitioners and health care facilities is the **numerical scale**. Patients are asked to rate their pain from zero to 10, with zero being no pain and 10 being the worst pain the patient can imagine. This is an effective tool when it is used consistently. Conventionally, the 1-4 range is considered mild pain; 5-6 is moderate pain; and 7-10 is severe pain. A question that can be asked in conjunction with this tool is "Are you satisfied with your current level of pain control?" Regardless of the numerical rating the patient assigns to the pain, a negative answer to this question should prompt additional efforts to relieve pain, while satisfaction with the current regimen allows continued observation.

Another commonly used scale is the **Wong-Baker FACES scale** (Hockenberry, Wilson, & Winkelstein, 2005):

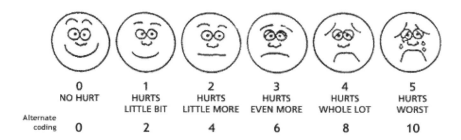

From Wong's *Essential Pediatric Nursing* (7th ed.) (p. 1259), by M. J. Hockenberry, D. Wilson, & M. L. Winkerstein, 2005, St. Louis, MO: Mosby. Copyright, Mosby. Used with permission.

The patient is asked to identify the face that best reflects how he or she is feeling. This scale has proven reliable for adults as well as children and has been used by clinicians observing the faces of patients who are unable to participate in the assessment process.

A physical examination can add valuable information to the historical data. In addition to the usual examination, performed according to good medical practice, attention should be focused on the area of pain. Tenderness, unusual skin sensitivity, and active and passive range of motion of affected limbs will contribute to the overall evaluation. Gait and posture can also reveal characteristics that suggest the nature of the pain. Neurological examination provides clues that will help clarify the nature of the pain and direct therapy.

DIAGNOSTIC TESTING

In an age of explosive development in medical technology, it is a challenge to avoid extensive workups in the midst of an evaluation for pain, but discretion is important. When the diagnosis is known, diagnostic testing (laboratory or imaging) only infrequently contributes meaningfully to the evaluative process. Certainly, if the cause of the pain is unknown, it is important to use every means to establish the diagnosis or condition and clarify the etiology. But testing should be reserved for circumstances in which the answer will establish the diagnosis or affect the treatment plan.

Psychosocial and Existential Considerations

One of the most important components of a comprehensive pain assessment is the psychosocial evaluation. To develop an effective therapeutic program, it is of critical importance to identify the presence of depression, anxiety, other psychiatric or psychological disorder, substance abuse, marital or other relational discord, or spiritual distress. Many people manifest existential or emotional distress through somatic pain, which may feel, look, and act like pain that has organic or physical disease roots. It is not uncommon for patients to undergo extensive testing and powerful treatment regimens for pain that is actually caused by unresolved grief, alcoholism, or depression overlooked in the earnest attempt to treat what looked like somatic disease-based pain. An additional challenge is that the very nature of chronic pain and the conditions that create pain can produce psychological distress. Patients have wished for death and even attempted suicide to be released from an unbearable burden of pain. This complex scenario requires aggressive psychosocial as well as medical intervention.

Impact of Pain on the Whole Person

Just as physical, psychosocial, and spiritual factors contribute to the symptom of pain, so can pain influence these components of the human condition. Indeed, pain leaves no domain of life untouched.

- The impact of pain on **physical well-being** and associated symptoms are the typical motivators for seeking medical attention. Functional ability and strength may be affected, with constitutional symptoms such as fatigue, insomnia, anorexia, nausea, and constipation also presenting. Preexisting symptoms may worsen in the presence of pain, as thresholds are lowered.

- **Psychological symptoms** such as anxiety and depression may develop as a result of chronic pain, as feelings of hopelessness, helplessness, and dependency manifest themselves. Fear is also a predominant factor. Patients may fear that increased pain means the disease is worsening. They also may believe that their complaints are perceived negatively by their provider. For example, they may fear that their physician will minimize the severity of their symptoms, accuse them of drug-seeking behaviors, or view them as difficult or complaining. All these emotional reactions can significantly erode a person's sense of psychological well-being. Leisure activities are typically curtailed in the face of significant pain, and cognition and attentive capabilities may be negatively affected.

- Patients may experience **spiritual angst** as they question the meaning of their pain, view it as a form of retribution or punishment, or feel that they have been abandoned by God in their time of need. Some patients may view their suffering as a necessary penance to achieve spiritual completeness.

- Pain also has a significant impact in the **social and relational** domain. Family roles are altered as pain prevents the patient from accomplishing usual tasks at home or at work. The impact (real or perceived) on physical appearance may result in social withdrawal and tension in relationships. Pain has a significant impact on sexual relationships, as well as nonsexual demonstrations of affection. Many patients who are experiencing functional impairment as a result of pain are very worried about the burden they are imposing on their primary caregiver, as well as the financial impact their condition may have on the family.

Before appropriate interventions and resources can be accessed for the patient experiencing pain, these domains must be considered and understood. Appropriately trained personnel (social workers, psychologists, and chaplains) should be engaged to help patients with pain issues that are affecting their daily functioning and psychospiritual well-being.

ADDITIONAL CONSIDERATIONS

- It is not unusual for a pain patient, especially one who has cancer, to have multiple foci of pain. It is important to elicit all that the patient may have to share about the variety of pains, to listen carefully, and to address each pain individually and completely.

- Patients with chronic debilitating conditions may also suffer from common ailments and discomforts from time to time, such as headache or back pain. It is important not to minimize these complaints, but to treat them appropriately. For example, a patient who is being treated with opioids for cancer-related pain can also be treated with typical mild analgesics for a non-cancer-related headache.

- Patient logs are invaluable in assessing the effectiveness of a prescribed regimen. Tracking the emergence of pain; its duration, response to medications, and impact on function; and other constitutional symptoms can be a meaningful way for patients to see firsthand the objective results of the plan of care. Patient logs also provide the practitioner with a reliable guide for adjusting therapy.

- Reassessment of pain and documentation of the patient response are essential for effective, ongoing pain management. Scheduling timely follow-up and monitoring the patient closely will optimize the opportunities for symptom relief and minimize the potential for side effects, as well as intentional or unintentional misuse or abuse of prescribed opioids. The failure of a patient to respond to typical types, dosages, and titration of opioid analgesics could suggest an unidentified pain focus, opioid tolerance, or drug misuse or diversion.

Summary

Albert Schweitzer once wrote, "We all must die. But if I can save him from days of torture, that is what I feel is my great and ever new privilege. Pain is a more terrible lord of mankind than even death itself" (Schweitzer, 1931, p. 62).

The medical community has a great opportunity to address and positively affect the ubiquitous prevalence of pain. To do so will require compassionate hearts and creative minds, confidence in the science of analgesia, and a commitment to eliminating suffering that is as passionate as the profession's commitment to the destruction of disease. We should be in the business of treating *people* rather than reflecting a model that emphasizes treating the *disease*. The challenge can be met, and we must start with an unqualified comprehensive assessment of those presenting with pain. ■

After working as a family physician for 17 years in Michigan, John Mulder, MD, moved to Nashville, TN, in the year 2000 to assume a full-time career in hospice and palliative medicine. He currently serves as Vice President of Clinical Services and Medical Director of Alive Hospice, based in Nashville. Additionally, he has an appointment as Assistant Professor in the Departments of Medicine and Pediatrics at the Vanderbilt University School of Medicine, teaching the next generation of physicians and nurse practitioners in the art and skill of end-of-life care. He serves as the Clinical Director of the Pain and Symptom Management Program at the Vanderbilt Ingram Cancer Center, and is sought after nationally as a speaker and authority on end of life issues as well as pain and symptom management.

Since 1990 he has served on the Board of Directors of International Aid, a relief and development agency and served as the organization's Chairman from 1995-2002. Dr. Mulder has also facilitated medical care and adoption for scores of children orphaned or abandoned in Eastern Europe. Finally, Dr. Mulder is involved in the musical arena, performing as a singer/songwriter in the folk genre around the world and recording five albums of his music.

Suggested Reading

Foley. K. M. (2004). Acute and chronic cancer pain syndromes. In D. Doyle, G. Hanks, N. Cherny, & K. Calman (Eds.), *Oxford textbook of palliative medicine* (pp. 298-314). New York: Oxford Medical Publications.

Health Care Association of New Jersey (HCANJ). (2005, January). *Pain management guidelines.* Hamilton, NJ: HCANJ.

Institute for Clinical Systems Improvement (ICSI). (2004, March). *Assessment and management of acute pain.* Bloomington, MN: ICSI.

Miaskowski, C., Cleary, J., Burney, R., Coyne, P., Finley, R., Foster, R., et al. (2005). *Guideline for the management of cancer pain in adults and children.* Glenview, IL: American Pain Society.

Wong, D., & Baker, C. (1988). Pain in children: Comparison of assessment scales. *Pediatric Nursing, 14*(1), 9-17.

Wisconsin Medical Society Task Force on Pain Management. (2004). Guidelines for the assessment and management of chronic pain. *Wisconsin Medical Journal,103*(3),13-42.

REFERENCES

McCaffery, M. (1968). *Nursing practice theories related to cognition, bodily pain, and man-environment interactions.* Los Angeles: University of California, Los Angeles Student Store.

Schweitzer A. (1931). *On the edge of the primeval forest.* New York: McMillan.

GUIDELINES FOR ASSESSING PAIN IN CULTURALLY DIVERSE POPULATIONS

It is critically important to remember that pain assessment is more complicated when working with a person whose cultural background is different from one's own. Each culture views pain from a unique vantage point. Some cultures, for example, may emphasize a fatalistic or stoic approach to pain. Different cultural groups have their own beliefs about how pain can be understood and treated.

- *Know your own attitudes and beliefs.* Culture hides from those who know it best. Each person has his or her own beliefs about pain and pain behaviors. How do your attitudes and beliefs about pain influence your response to individuals from other cultures? For example, do you admire those who stoically bear pain without complaint? Do you hold any attitudes or suspicions that persons from certain groups or social classes might abuse pain medications? Begin by being aware of your own biases and beliefs.

- *Develop a relationship with your patients.* Effective pain assessment is more likely to occur in an atmosphere in which patients trust health professionals and believe that their concerns and perspectives are being listened to, validated, and valued. Remember that people who have experienced social discrimination and prejudice in the past may need more time to develop trust.

- *Assess patients' cultural beliefs and practices regarding pain.* Be open to learning about other cultures. The question "What do I need to understand about your cultural background to effectively treat you?" not only provides information about the patient's culture; it also communicates an attitude of respect and concern. Assessing a patient's beliefs and practices allows you to determine whether any barriers exist that might inhibit effective pain management. For example, the fatalism of some cultural groups may create a feeling that pain is inevitable and should be borne without complaint.

■ *Use cultural practices and folk remedies when possible as complementary aspects of treatment.* Determine what members of the patient's cultural group generally do to relieve pain. When possible, incorporate these practices into the treatment plan. People are more likely to adhere to a medical regimen that reflects their cultural beliefs and practices.

■ *Self-report is one of the most reliable tools of pain assessment.* Use the Wong-Baker FACES pain rating scale or a numerical (0 to 10) scale such the Oucher scale to rate pain. African-American and Hispanic versions of the Oucher scale are available. Translate scales into the languages of patients if English is not their primary language.

■ *Ask "Are you comfortable?" rather than "Are you in pain?"* In certain cultures, it is unseemly to complain about pain. Asking about comfort is a more comprehensive way to assess a patient's condition and is less likely to elicit a defensive response.

■ *Use a family-centered approach.* Involving the family in pain assessment and management will help ensure adherence, especially in Hispanic/Latino, Native American, and Asian cultures, which are typically very family-centered.

■ *Make sure instructions for medications are clearly understood.* It is helpful to provide directions in the patient's language of choice and to make sure that the patient, family members, and others in the person's support network clearly understand the directions.

■ *If you use a translator, talk with the translator about the approach he or she takes in communicating information.* Each culture has different norms about what can or cannot be comfortably communicated. For example, in some cultures, the translator may feel compelled to soften "bad news" or may be embarrassed to ask certain personal questions. It is best that such constraints are understood and discussed before you attempt to communicate with the patient.

continued

- ***Use preventive analgesics to keep pain ratings at an acceptable level.***
  Patients are more likely to trust the health care provider and feel less fatalistic
  about pain when they perceive that the provider is doing everything possible
  and when their pain is kept at an acceptable level.

Each person has numerous cultural identities—we are defined not only by ethnicity
and race but also by social class, lifestyle, spirituality, and geography. You can never
assume that you know your patient's full cultural identity. Effective pain assessment
and management for culturally diverse populations is, in the final analysis, simply
good pain assessment and management.

—Kenneth J. Doka, PhD

CHAPTER 6

Older Adults With Severe Cognitive Impairment: Assessment of Pain

By Keela Herr and Sheila Decker

Revised and reprinted from
Annals of Long-Term Care: Clinical Care and Aging 2004; 12(4):46-52

Despite the prevalence and consequences of pain among older adults, pain is inadequately recognized and treated, especially in those with severe cognitive impairment. Among the barriers to assessment of pain in this challenging population are the inability of some older patients to communicate their pain experience and the misconception that pain is less severe in those with cognitive impairment.

Although continued research is needed to evolve the evidence for best practices, current guidelines and research can provide recommendations to improve assessment practices when caring for this vulnerable population. Use of surrogate reporters, direct observation of potential pain indicators, monitoring for changes in baseline activity patterns, and ruling pain out as a possible cause of behaviors through nondrug and analgesic trials are identified as key elements of an approach to assessing pain in those with severe cognitive impairment.

INTRODUCTION

More than 1.5 million Americans live in nursing homes, a number that will dramatically increase in the next two decades, and up to 80% of long-term care facility residents experience substantial pain (Baer & Hanson, 2000; Ferrell, Ferrell, & Rivera, 1995; Won, Lapane, Vallow, Schein, Morris, et al., 2004). Because pain is often remediable (American Geriatrics Society (AGS), 2002), it is thought that the high prevalence estimates of unrelieved pain in older persons may result from underrecognition, which in turn results in undertreatment (Horgas & Tsai, 1998; Morrison & Siu, 2000; Weiner, Peterson, Ladd, McConnell, & Keefe, 1999). Unrecognized and thus untreated (or undertreated) pain can have serious consequences for the quality of life of older persons. Unrelieved pain has been associated with altered immune function, impaired psychological function (e.g., depression, anxiety, fear), impaired physical function (e.g., impaired mobility and gait, delayed rehabilitation, falls), sleep disturbance, compromised cognitive function, and decreased socialization (AGS, 2002; Brummel-Smith, London, Drew, Krulewitch, Singer. et al., 2002; Hartikainen, Mantyselka, Louhivuori-Laako, & Sulkava, 2005; Herrick et al., 2004; Jakobsson, Rahm Hallberg, & Westergren, 2004; Landi et al., 2005; Schuler, Njoo, Hestermann, Oster, & Hauer, 2004; Weiner, Herr, & Rudy, 2002). These negative consequences can result in increased dependency and helplessness, as well as increased use of health care resources, and eventually in increased costs. In those with severe cognitive impairment, these outcomes are often attributed to other conditions, such as dementia, rather than to unrecognized and untreated painful conditions. The ultimate impact of pain on quality of life in this population is difficult to determine (Brummel-Smith et al., 2002).

Despite the prevalence and consequences of pain among older adults, health care professionals remain ineffective at both its assessment (Hall-Lord, Larrson, & Steen, 1998; Herr et al., 2004; Weiner, Peterson, & Keefe, 1999) and its treatment (Bernabei et al., 1998; Morrison & Siu, 2000; Teno, Weitzen, Wetle, & Mor, 2001; 2004; Won et al., 2004), especially in those who are unable to communicate their discomfort. Older adults with cognitive impairment receive less pain medication than those who are able to communicate, even though they are just as likely to experience painful illnesses. Studies have also shown that those with more disorientation and functional impairment receive fewer analgesics (Feldt, Ryden, & Miles, 1998; Horgas & Tsai, 1998; Morrison & Siu, 2000; Won et al., 2004). Multiple factors contribute to poor pain management in this population; however, the most troublesome is the failure to recognize pain in elders who cannot communicate their pain experience (Herr, Bjoro, & Decker, in press). Therefore, it is imperative that health care professionals' knowledge and skills related to pain assessment in older adults be improved and aggressive approaches to comprehensive pain assessment be adopted.

BARRIERS TO PAIN ASSESSMENT IN OLDER ADULTS WITH SEVERE COGNITIVE IMPAIRMENT

Awareness of barriers that interfere with effective assessment and management of pain is important in developing a plan of care that promotes comfort in the older adult. The most obvious barrier is the inability of the person with severe dementia to communicate the presence of pain, at least in a manner that is easily understood, and to assist in the differentiation of pain etiologies. This necessitates alternative approaches to assessment in this population, which are discussed below.

Although a number of misconceptions and fears have been commonly identified in older adults (Herr & Garand, 2001), it is the misconceptions and lack of knowledge of the patient's family/significant other and the health care provider that must be addressed in order to provide quality pain assessment and intervention to patients with severe cognitive impairment. A major misconception that affects recognition of pain in this population is the belief that cognitively impaired older adults do not experience pain as severely as those who are intact. There is no convincing evidence that peripheral nociceptor responses or pain transmission are impaired in people with dementia, although controversy does exist about central nervous system changes that influence or diminish interpretation of pain transmission (Gibson, Voukelatos, Ames, Flicker, & Helme, 2001; Scherder, Slaets, Deijen, Gorter, Ooms, al., 2003; Schuler et al., 2004). People with dementia may have altered affective responses to pain, probably due to their inability to cognitively process the painful sensation in the context of prior pain experience, attitudes, knowledge, and beliefs

(Scherder, Oosterman, Swaab, Herr, Ooms et al., 2005). Reactions to painful sensations may differ from the typical response expected from a cognitively intact older person. For example, constipation can cause great distress in the cognitively impaired older patient and may lead to aggressive or agitated behaviors. Thus, until evidence establishes that those with dementia experience less pain, we should assume that any condition that is painful to a cognitively intact person would also be painful to those with advanced dementia who cannot express themselves. This assumption has implications for the recognition and management of pain in this population. Knowledge of possible indicators of pain presence in the older adult with severe cognitive impairment and strategies for assessment are key. Integration of content into health care that provides curricula, continuing education for current providers, and family/caregiver education is essential.

ASSESSMENT APPROACHES FOR OLDER PERSONS WITH SEVERE COGNITIVE IMPAIRMENT

The AGS Panel on Persistent Pain (2002) and the American Medical Directors Association (2003) have developed guidelines to address the needs of older adults with persistent pain in a variety of settings. These guidelines provide assistance to clinicians with decision-making responsibilities regarding pain assessment and management in older persons, although additional research is needed to further refine recommendations related to those with severe cognitive impairment. Figure 1 presents a practical approach to evaluating the presence of pain in the nonverbal cognitively impaired older patient (Reuben et al., 2005).

While evidence exists that older adults with cognitive impairment can complete self-report pain scales (Chibnall & Tait, 2001; Closs, Barr, Briggs, Cash, & Seers, 2004; Herr, Spratt, Mobily, & Richardson, 2004; Kaasalainen & Crook, 2003; Scherder et al., 2003; Taylor & Herr, 2003; Taylor, Harris, Epps, & Herr, 2005), a challenge remains in assessing pain in older adults who experience more severe cognitive decline associated with a loss of language skills. Whereas self-report of pain is the gold standard for pain assessment, other approaches are necessary in this population, such as observational and surrogate reports. Although a precise and accurate method for interpreting the expression of pain in persons with cognitive

FIGURE 1. ALGORITHM FOR THE ASSESSMENT OF PAIN IN ELDERS WITH SEVERE COGNITIVE IMPAIRMENT

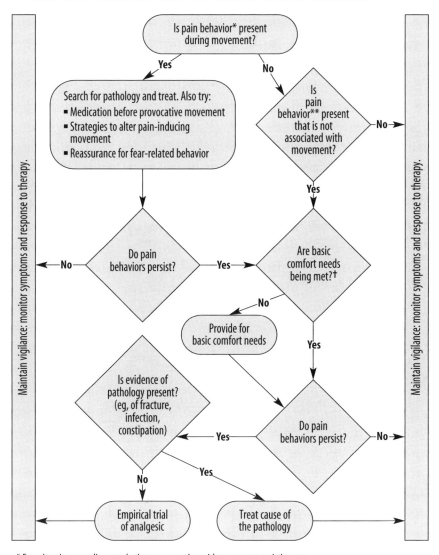

* Eg, grimacing, guarding, combativeness, groaning with movement; resisting care.
** Eg, agitation, fidgeting, sleep disturbance, diminished appetite, irritability, reclusiveness, disruptive behavior, rigidity, rapid blinking.
† Eg, toileting, thirst, hunger, visual or hearing impairment.

Note. From Reuben, DB, Herr, KA, Pacala JT, et al. *Geriatrics At Your Fingertips: 2005,* 7th Edition, p. 142. The American Geriatrics Society; 2005. Used with permission.

impairment is not available, recommendations can be made to guide practice decisions and provide a framework to guide future research in this important area.

DIRECT OBSERVATION: SURROGATE REPORTERS

When older patients are unable to use traditional self-report pain instruments, direct observation by health care providers and eliciting information from surrogates (family members, aides) is essential (AGS, 2002). It can be difficult to recognize that certain behaviors may indicate pain if the health care provider is unfamiliar with how the person usually behaves. Caregivers can be very helpful in recognizing changes in persons with dementia that might indicate pain. Caregivers with the most direct and long-standing relationship with the patient are in the best position to recognize subtle changes and communicate them to the health care provider (Cohen-Mansfield & Creedon, 2002). However, surrogate reporters must have preparation and training regarding the types of behaviors and activity changes that might indicate pain.

Although studies of pain behavior observation protocols suggest that well-trained surrogate ratings of pain are relatively accurate (Dirks, Wunder, Kingsman, McElhinny, & Jones, 1993; Richards, Nepomuceno, Riles, & Suer, 1982; Weiner, Peterson, & Keefe, 1999), outcomes for health care and family surrogates are much more disappointing. When patient self-reported pain ratings are compared with those of professional caregivers (health care surrogates), both physicians and nurses tend to underestimate the severity of the patient's pain (Cohen-Mansfield & Lipson, 2002; Fisher et al., 2002; Hall-Lord et al., 1998; Horgas & Dunn, 2001; Weiner, Peterson, & Keefe, 1999). While family caregivers are more adept at estimating the pain of others, they tend to overestimate the intensity of pain (Cohen-Mansfield, 2002; Yeager, Miaskowski, Dibble, & Wallhagen, 1995). Although surrogate reporters have difficulty accurately identifying the severity of pain from behavioral observation, they are able to recognize the presence of pain (Manfredi, Breuer, Meier, & Libow, 2003; Shega, Hougham, Stocking, Cox-Hayley, & Sachs, 2004). Certified nursing assistants (CNAs) are more familiar with residents, can identify pain in this population, and play an important role in recognizing pain (Closs, Cash,

Barr, & Briggs, 2005; Fisher et al., 2002; Mentes, Teer, & Cadogan, 2004). Clearly, further investigative efforts are needed to refine the process of surrogate pain rating. However, until a more reliable method of detecting pain in noncommunicative older patients is determined, direct observation of patient behavior and surrogate reporting of pain are essential in our efforts to determine the presence of pain in this population.

PAIN INDICATORS: NONVERBAL CUES AND CHANGES IN USUAL ACTIVITY

Because most persons with advanced dementia are unable to verbally report their pain experience, observation of behaviors and activities that may indicate pain is a key assessment strategy. Caregivers should be alert for the presence of typical pain behaviors, as well as those that are less obvious and not usually attributed to pain. Table 1 includes a detailed list of common behaviors of cognitively impaired older adults who are in pain (AGS, 2002). Table 2 provides take-home pearls regarding the assessment of pain in this challenging population. Some typical pain behaviors are rubbing, guarding, moaning, groaning, crying, grimacing, and frowning. In noncommunicative older adults with severe cognitive impairment, common pain behaviors may be absent or difficult to interpret, and it is important to be alert for less obvious potential indicators of pain. For example, some forms of dementia tend to mute facial expression, while other forms of dementia appear not to affect facial expressions at all (Asplund, Norberg, Adolfssonm, & Waxman, 1991). Also, agitation and disturbing or aggressive behaviors attributed to dementia actually may be indicators of pain (Buffum, Miaskowski, Sands, & Brod, 2001; Kovach, Noonan, Griffie, Muchka, & Weissman, 2001). Observation for pain behaviors at rest can be misleading, with increased indicators of pain observed during activities such as transferring, ambulating, and reposi-tioning (Feldt, 2000; Feldt, Ryden & Miles, 1998; Hadjistavropolous, LaChapelle, MacLeod, Snider, & Craig, 2000; Weiner, Pieper, McConnell, Martinez & Keefe, 1996). Thus, observation for indicators of pain should include active times.

More subtle and less specific nonverbal indicators of pain may include facial expressions (e.g., distorted expressions, rapid blinking,

TABLE 1. COMMON PAIN BEHAVIORS IN COGNITIVELY IMPAIRED ELDERLY PERSONS

Facial expressions

- Slight frown; sad, frightened face
- Grimacing, wrinkled forehead; closed or tightened eyes
- Any distorted expression
- Rapid blinking

Verbalizations and vocalizations

- Sighing, moaning, groaning
- Grunting, chanting, calling out
- Noisy breathing
- Asking for help
- Verbally abusive

Body movements

- Rigid, tense body posture
- Guarding
- Fidgeting
- Increased pacing, rocking
- Restricted movement
- Gait or mobility changes

Changes in interpersonal interactions

- Refusing food, appetite change
- Increase in rest periods
- Sleep/rest pattern changes
- Sudden cessation of common routines
- Increased wandering

Mental status changes

- Crying or tears
- Increased confusion
- Irritability or distress

Note. Some patients demonstrate little or no specific behavior associated with severe pain. From "The management of persistent pain in older persons," by the American Geriatrics Society Panel on Persistent Pain in Older Persons, 2002, *Journal of the American Geriatrics Society, 50,* pp. S205-S224. Used with permission.

frightened face); verbalizations/vocalizations (e.g., grunting, chanting, verbally abusive, yelling out); body movements (e.g., fidgeting, increased pacing or rocking, rigid posture); changes in interpersonal interactions (e.g., aggressive, resisting care, disruptive, withdrawn); changes in activity patterns or routines (e.g., sudden cessation of common routines, refusing food, increased sleep, increased wandering); and mental status changes (e.g., increased confusion, irritability, distress) (Table 2) (AGS, 2002; Closs et al., 2005; Cohen-Mansfield & Creedon, 2002; Fuchs-Lacelle & Hadjistavropolous, 2004; Hadjistavropolous & Craig, 2002; Kovach, Weissmann, Griffie, Matson, & Muchka, 1999; Manfredi, Breuer, Meier, Libow, 2003). Establishing the individual's typical or baseline pattern of behavior and activity is essential in being able to recognize changes that may reflect unrecognized pain problems. For example, pain should be considered as one potential etiology if the older person with advanced dementia shows decreased activity or increased activity, change in appetite or intake, change in mood, increased agitation or restlessness, increased pacing or wandering, combativeness or aggressive behaviors, withdrawal or isolation, or increase in verbal outbursts/screaming. Although subtle changes in usual patterns of behavior or activity do not always mean that the patient is in pain, they raise the suspicion and should lead to thorough evaluation for possible pain-causing problems.

BEHAVIORAL PAIN TOOLS

Persons with cognitive impairment present with a unique "pain signature." Whereas one patient may become withdrawn and quiet, another may become agitated. Both of these behavior patterns could indicate pain, but they are difficult to reconcile with behavioral tools that attempt to score behaviors by pain intensity and that are narrow in the indicators included. In an effort to enhance the validity and reliability of behaviors for quantifying pain in older adults with severe cognitive impairment, assessment approaches that focus on behavioral observation are being developed and evaluated. Tools and approaches most readily recognized in the literature include the Discomfort in Dementia of the Alzheimer's Type (DS-DAT) (Hurley, Volicer, Hanrahan, Houde, & Volicer, 1992), the Modified DS-DAT (Miller et al., 1996); the Checklist of Nonverbal Pain

Indicators (CNPI) (Feldt, 2000); and the Assessment of Discomfort in Dementia (ADD) Protocol (Kovach, Noonan, Griffie, Muchka, & Weissman, 2002). In addition, several other tools are available to assess pain in this population, including the Pain Assessment in Advanced Dementia (PAINAD) scale (Warden, Hurley, & Volicer, 2003); the Nursing Assistant-Administered Instrument to Assess Pain in Demented Individuals (NOPPAIN) (Snow, Weber, O'Malley, Cody, Beck, 2004) and the Pain Assessment Checklist for Seniors with Severe Dementia (PACSLAC) (Fuchs-Lacelle & Hadjistravropolous, 2004). Several promising approaches to behavioral assessment in the nonverbal, cognitively impaired older adult exist, but most are in the early stages of testing or are limited in their clinical utility. These tools and approaches have various strengths and limitations related to the available evidence to support their use in clinical practice. A state-of-the-science review of available nonverbal assessment tools is available to guide the clinician in selecting a tool appropriate for the patient and setting (Herr, Bjoro & Decker) in press).

The testing of existing behavioral observation assessment instruments in minority older adults with dementia is limited. With an increase in cultural diversity in the United States (Administration on Aging, 2003; Hayward & Zhang, 2001); an increase in dementia among minority populations (Alzheimer's Disease International, 1999); and evidence that minority patients are undertreated (Bernabei et al., 1998; Teno, Kabunoto, Wetle, Roy, & Mor, 2004; Won, Lapene, Gambassi, Bernabei, Mor, et al., 1999), it is important for researchers to extend development and evaluation of observational assessment tools to address minority older adults with dementia.

SEARCH FOR CAUSES OF PAIN/DISCOMFORT

If pain behaviors or activity changes are observed, the practitioner should attempt to determine whether pain is the etiology, as many of these nonspecific behaviors (e.g., agitation, restlessness, yelling, withdrawal, pacing) could be related to other causes or to the disease process of dementia. When pain is suspected, a search for possible causes is important to guide treatment decisions. Common problems (e.g., constipation, inflammation, infection, fractures, pressure ulcers) or procedures

TABLE 2. TAKE-HOME PEARLS

1. Health care providers and caregivers/families often harbor myths and misconceptions about pain and its treatment in the nonverbal elder with severe cognitive impairment that must be recognized and debunked.

2. The most common reason that pain is undertreated in older adults is failure to assess it.

3. Older persons often have multiple persistent pain problems that must be considered in evaluation of new and ongoing pain conditions.

4. Alternative strategies are important when assessing pain in older persons who cannot communicate their pain.

5. Subtle pain behaviors or changes in routine/activities may be indicators of the presence of pain in those with severe cognitive impairment.

6. If behavioral changes are noted, assume that pain is present until proven otherwise.

7. If you would experience pain in similar circumstances, assume that the nonverbal cognitively impaired person would as well.

8. Use of pain treatments (e.g., pharmacologic and nonpharmacologic approaches) plays a key role in evaluating for the presence of pain in persons who cannot communicate.

9. Involvement of family and/or caregivers may be useful in recognizing changes in behavior/activities that may suggest the presence of pain.

10. Teach family members and caregivers about the relationship between behavioral and activity changes and pain to facilitate their help in pain assessment.

11. Regular reassessment is essential to evaluate and monitor response to pain interventions and to recognize the return of pain or new pain problems.

12. The same scale and behavioral manifestations used to identify pain in older persons should be used in evaluating the effectiveness of interventions.

13. Identified pain behaviors (specific and nonspecific) must be communicated to other health care providers and across care settings.

Source: Keela Herr and Sheila Decker

(e.g., dressing changes) that are known to be uncomfortable should be considered as possible causes of changes in behavior (Morrison, Ahron-heim, Morrison, Darling, Baskin, et al., 1998). A number of chronic pain problems prevalent in older adults should be considered when exploring possible pain etiologies. For example, up to 80% of older adults experience osteoarthritis, so this is a common reason for pain in this population. Other conditions that should be considered are inflammatory arthritis, neuralgias (e.g., postherpetic neuralgia, trigeminal neuralgia), peripheral neuropathy (ischemic and diabetic), temporal arteritis and polymyalgia rheumatica, osteoporosis-related compression fractures, low back pain, spinal stenosis, old and undiagnosed fractures, myofascial pain syndromes, post-stroke syndrome, phantom limb pain, and many types of cancer (Donald & Foy, 2004; Weiner & Herr, 2002). If the patient has a disease that would be painful to others who can verbalize, assume that it is painful for the person with advanced dementia. Efforts should focus on treating any identifiable pathologies and premedicating before painful procedures. If physical causes are ruled out, interventions should focus on basic comfort measures (such as positioning, toileting, soothing communication, addressing hunger and thirst, managing environmental stimuli) and addressing unmet needs (Kovach et al., 2002; Miller et al., 1996). Sources of environmental stress (e.g., loud noises, glare from lights, poorly fitting clothes or shoes), balance between rest and activity, and level of human interaction should be considered (Kovach et al., 2002).

ANALGESIC TRIAL

If pain behaviors continue after other possible causes are ruled out or treated, an empiric analgesic trial is warranted as an assessment approach. Because it is difficult to determine the level of pain severity in persons with advanced dementia, selection of an appropriate analgesic is challenging. The few studies that have examined use of an analgesic trial start with a nonopioid such as acetaminophen 500-1000 mg three times a day (Buffum, Sands, Miaskowski, Brod, & Washburn, 2004; Douzjian et al., 1998; Kovach et al., 1999; 2002). However, titration to higher doses and stronger analgesics may be necessary before ruling out pain as the etiology for behavior or activity changes (Manfredi, Breuer, Wallenstein et al., 2003).

If interventions appear to result in pain relief (e.g., decreased agitation or restlessness), assume that pain was the likely cause and continue pharmacologic and/or nonpharmacologic interventions. If behavioral changes persist or intensify, continue to rule out and focus treatment on other possible causes, such as delirium, adverse effects of treatment, and drug metabolite accumulation.

Preliminary research on the use of an analgesic trial as part of the protocol for assessing the presence of pain in the noncommunicative older adult suggests that this approach can reduce pain-related behaviors (Kovach et al., 2002; Manfredi, Breuer, Meier et al., 2003), although further research in controlled studies is needed to develop an algorithm to guide practice decisions.

REASSESSMENT AND COMMUNICATION STRATEGIES

Reassessment of pain and other symptoms, using the same assessment approach, should be conducted at regular intervals at times that relate to the anticipated peak and duration of administered analgesics. Because recognition of subtle changes in behavior is difficult for anyone without an ongoing history/knowledge of the individual patient's usual behavior pattern, any specific behaviors or activity changes that are being monitored must be communicated to other health care providers and caregivers to ensure continuity of care when the older person with severe cognitive impairment is moving between care providers or care settings. Development of a transfer document or communication approach (e.g., faxed information sheet) that incorporates this individualized assessment would be helpful to ensure communication of essential information.

SUMMARY

Although the science to guide pain assessment practices in older adults with severe cognitive impairment is still evolving, adopting current recommendations for practice should improve the recognition of pain in this vulnerable population. Interventions adapted to meet the needs of frail older adults must follow to improve comfort and quality of life for these elders in their final stage of life. ■

Keela Herr, PhD, RN, is Professor and Chair of Adult and Gerontological Nursing in the College of Nursing at the University of Iowa, Academic Associate in the Department of Nursing Services and Patient Care, University of Iowa Hospitals & Clinics in Iowa City, Research Director for the Iowa Hartford Center of Geriatric Nursing Excellence, and on the Steering Committee for the Geriatric Nursing Intervention Research Center at Iowa. She was recently appointed as Visiting Professor at Southern Medical University in Guangzhou, China from 2005-2007.

Over the past 17 years, Dr. Herr has been engaged in a program of research and scholarly and professional activities that has focused on the problem of pain in older adults. Dr. Herr recently completed service on the Board of Directors for the American Society for Pain Management Nursing and the American Pain Society and is currently on the Board of Directors of the American Geriatrics Society.

Sheila Decker earned her PhD in nursing from Saint Louis University, St. Louis, MO, and is a certified Gerontology Nurse Practitioner. Dr. Decker currently holds a faculty position as an Assistant Professor in the School of Nursing at The University of Texas Health Science Center-Houston. Her research interest is pain assessment and management in the elderly with dementia. She developed the Pain Assessment Tool in Confused Older Adults (PATCOA) to assess postoperative pain. Dr. Decker continues to conduct research in the area of instrument development to evaluate an instrument to assess persistent pain in elderly nursing home residents, and is extending that work to include minority elders with dementia. Her research in the area of pain management includes an interest in healing touch and massage therapy.

REFERENCES

Administration on Aging. (2003). *A profile of older Americans.* Washington, DC: Author.

American Geriatrics Society Panel on Persistent Pain in Older Persons. (2002). Clinical practice guidelines: The management of persistent pain in older persons. *Journal of the American Geriatrics Society, 50,* S205-S224.

Alzheimer's Disease International. (1999). *The prevalence of dementia.* London: Author.

American Medical Directors Association. (2003). *Chronic pain management in the long-term care setting—clinical practice guideline.* Author.

Asplund, K., Norberg, A., Adolfssonm, R., & Waxman, H. M. (1991). Facial expressions in severely demented patients: A stimulus-response study of four patients with dementia of the Alzheimer's type. *International Journal of Geriatric Psychiatry, 6,* 599-606.

Baer, W. M., & Hanson, L. C. (2000). Families' perception of the added value of hospice in the nursing home. *Journal of the American Geriatrics Society, 48*(8), 879-882.

Bernabei, R., Gambassi, G., Lapane, K., Landi, F., Gastonis, C., Dunlop, R., Lipsitz, L., Steel, K., & Mor, V., for the SAGE Study Group. (1998). Management of pain in elderly patients with cancer. *Journal of the American Medical Association, 279*(23), 1877-1882.

Brummel-Smith, K., London, M. R., Drew, N., Krulewitch, H., Singer, C., & Hanson, L. (2002). Outcomes of pain in frail older adults with dementia. *Journal of the American Geriatrics Society, 50*(11), 1847-1851.

Buffum, M., Miaskowski, C., Sands, L., & Brod, M. (2001). A pilot study of the relationship between discomfort and agitation in patients with dementia. *Geriatric Nursing, 22*(2), 80-85.

Buffum, M., Sands, L., Miaskowski, C., Brod, M., & Washburn, A. (2004). A clinical trial of the effectiveness of regularly scheduled versus as-needed administration of acetaminophen in the management of discomfort in older adults with dementia. *Journal of the American Geriatrics Society, 52,* 1093-1097.

Chibnall, J., & Tait, R. (2001). Pain assessment in cognitively impaired and unimpaired older adults: A comparison of four scales. *Pain, 92,* 173-186.

Closs, S. J., Barr, B., Briggs, M., Cash, K., & Seers, K. (2004). A comparison of five pain assessment scales for nursing home residents with varying degrees of cognitive impairment. *Journal of Pain and Symptom Management, 27*(3), 196-204.

Closs, S. J., Cash, K., Barr, B., & Briggs, M. (2005). Cues for the identification of pain in nursing home residents. *International Journal of Nursing Studies, 42*, 3-12.

Cohen-Mansfield, J. (2002). Relatives' assessment of pain in cognitively impaired nursing home residents. *Journal of Pain and Symptom Management, 4*(6), 562-571.

Cohen-Mansfield, J., & Creedon, M. (2002). Nursing staff members' perceptions of pain indicators in persons with severe dementia. *Clinical Journal of Pain, 18*(1), 64-73.

Cohen-Mansfield, J., & Lipson, S. (2002). Pain in cognitively impaired nursing home residents: How well are physicians diagnosing it? *Journal of the American Geriatrics Society, 50*, 1039-1044.

Dirks, J. F., Wunder, J., Kingsman, R., McElhinny, J., & Jones, N.F. (1993). A pain rating scale and pain behavior checklist for clinical use: Development, norms, and the consistency score. *Psychotherapy and Psychosomatics, 59*, 41-49.

Donald, I. P., & Foy, C. (2004). A longitudinal study of joint pain in older people. *Rheumatology, 43*(10), 1256-1260.

Douzjian, M., Wilson, C., Shultz, M., Berger, J., Tapnio, J., & Blanton, V. (1998). A program to use pain control medication to reduce psychotropic drug use in residents with difficult behavior. *Annals of Long Term Care, 6*(5), 174-179.

Feldt, K. S., Ryden, M. B., & Miles, S. (1998). Treatment of pain in cognitively impaired compared with cognitively intact older patients with hip fracture. *Journal of the American Geriatrics Society, 46*(9), 1079-1085.

Feldt, K. S. (2000). The Checklist of Nonverbal Pain Indicators (CNPI). *Pain Management Nursing, 1*(1), 13-21.

Ferrell, B. A., Ferrell, B. R., & Rivera, L. (1995). Pain in cognitively impaired nursing home patients. *Journal of Pain and Symptom Management, 10*, 591-598.

Fisher, S., Burgio, L., Thorn, B., Allen-Burge, R., Gerstle, J., Roth, D., & Allen, S. (2002). Pain assessment and management in cognitively impaired nursing home residents: Association of certified nursing assistant pain report, minimum data set pain report, and analgesic use. *Journal of the American Geriatrics Society, 50*(1), 152-156.

Fuchs-Lacelle, S., & Hadjistavropolous, T. (2004). Development and preliminary validation of the Pain Assessment Checklist for Seniors with Limited Ability to Communicate (PACSLAC). *Pain Management Nursing, 5*(1), 37-49.

Gibson, S., Voukelatos, X., Ames, D., Flicker, L., & Helme, R. (2001). An examination of pain perception and cerebral event-related potentials following carbon dioxide laser stimulation in patients with Alzheimer's disease and age-matched control volunteers. *Pain Research and Management, 6*(3), 126-132.

Hadjistavropolous, T., & Craig, K. (2002). A theoretical framework for understanding self-report and observational measures of pain: A communications model. *Behavior Research and Therapy, 40*(5), 551-570.

Hadjistravropolous, T., LaChapelle, D., MacLeod, F., Snider, B., & Craig, K. (2000). Measuring movement-exacerbated pain in cognitively impaired frail elders. *Clinical Journal of Pain, 16*(1), 54-63.

Hall-Lord, M. L., Larrson, G., & Steen, B. (1998). Pain and distress among elderly intensive care unit patients: Comparison of patients' experiences and nurses' assessments. *Heart and Lung, 27*(2), 123-132.

Hartikainen, S. A., Mantyselka, P. T., Louhivuori-Laako, K. A., & Sulkava, R. O. (2005). Balancing pain and analgesic treatment in the home-dwelling elderly. *Annals of Pharmacotherapy, 39*(1), 11-16.

Hayward, M. D., & Zhang, Z. (2001). Demography of aging: A century of global change, 1950-2050. In R. H. Binstock & L. K. George (Eds.), *Handbook of aging and the social sciences* (5th ed., pp. 69-85). San Diego, CA: Academic Press.

Herr, K., Bjoro, K., & Decker, S. (in press). A state-of-the-science review of nonverbal pain assessment tools for use in patients with dementia. *Journal of Pain and Symptom Management.*

Herr, K., & Garand, L. (2001). Assessment and measurement of pain in older adults. *Clinics in Geriatric Medicine, 17*(3), 457-478.

Herr, K., Spratt, K., Mobily, P., & Richardson, G. (2004). Pain intensity assessment in older adults: Use of experimental pain to compare psychometric properties and usability of selected scales with younger adults. *Clinical Journal of Pain, 20*(4), 207-219.

Herr, K. Titler, M., Schilling, M., Marsh, J. L., Xie, X., Ardery, G., et al. (2004). Evidence-based assessment of acute pain in older adults: Current nursing practices and perceived barriers. *Clinical Journal of Pain, 20*(5), 331-334.

Herrick, C., Steger-May, K., Sinacore, D. R., Brown, M., Schechtman, K. B., & Binder, E. F. (2004). Persistent pain in frail older adults after hip fracture repair. *Journal of the American Geriatrics Society, 52*(12), 2062-2068.

Horgas, A. L., & Dunn, K. (2001). Pain in nursing home residents: Comparison of residents' self-report and nursing assistants' perceptions. *Journal of Gerontological Nursing, 27*(3), 44-53.

Horgas, A. L., & Tsai, P. F. (1998). Analgesic drug prescription and use in cognitively impaired nursing home residents. *Nursing Research, 47*, 235-242.

Hurley, A. C., Volicer, B. J., Hanrahan, P. A., Houde, S., & Volicer, L. (1992). Assessment of discomfort in advanced Alzheimer's patients. *Research in Nursing and Health Care, 15*(5), 369-377.

Jakobsson, W., Rahm Hallberg, I., & Westergren, A. (2004). Pain management in elderly persons who require assistance with activities of daily living: A comparison of those living at home with those in special accommodations. *European Journal of Pain, 8*(4), 335-344.

Kaasalainen, S., & Crook, J. (2003). A comparison of pain-assessment tools for use with elderly long-term-care residents. *Clinical Journal of Nursing Research, 35*(4), 58-71.

Kovach, C., Noonan, P., Griffie, J., Muchka, S., & Weissman, D. (2002). The assessment of discomfort in dementia protocol. *Pain Management Nursing, 3*(1), 16-27.

Kovach, C., Noonan, P., Griffie, J., Muchka, S., & Weissman, D. (2001). Use of the assessment of Ddiscomfort in dementia protocol. *Applied Nursing Research, 14*(4), 193-200.

Kovach, C. R., Weissman, D. E., Griffie, J., Matson, S., & Muchka, S. (1999). Assessment and treatment of discomfort for people with late-stage dementia. *Journal of Pain and Symptom Management, 18*(6), 291-294.

Landi, F., Onder, G., Cesari, M., Russo, A., Barillaro, C., & Bernabei, R. (2005). Pain and its relation to depressive symptoms in frail older people living in the community: An observational study. *Journal of Pain and Symptom Management, 29*(3), 255-262.

Manfredi, P., Breuer, B., Meier, D., & Libow, L. (2003). Pain assessment in elderly patients with severe dementia. *Journal of Pain and Symptom Management, 25*(1), 48-52.

Manfredi, P., Breuer, B., Wallenstein, S., Stegmann, M., Bottomley, G., & Libow, L. (2003). Opioid treatment for agitation in patients with advanced dementia. *International Journal of Geriatric Psychiatry, 18*, 700-705.

Mentes, J. C., Teer, J., & Cadogan, M. P. (2004). The pain experience of cognitively impaired nursing home residents: Perceptions of family members and certified nursing assistants. *Pain Management Nursing, 5*(3), 118-125.

Miller, J., Neelon, V., Dalton, J., Ng'andu, N., Bailey, D., Jr., Layman, E., & Hosfeld, A. (1996). The assessment of discomfort in elderly confused patients: A preliminary study. *Journal of Neuroscience Nursing, 28*, 175-182.

Morrison, R. S., Ahronheim, J. C., Morrison, G. R., Darling, E., Baskin, S. A., Morris, J., et al. (1998). Pain and discomfort associated with common hospital procedures and experiences. *Journal of Pain and Symptom Management, 15*(2), 91-101.

Morrison, R. S., & Siu, A. L. (2000). A comparison of pain and its treatment in advanced dementia and cognitively intact patients with hip fracture. *Journal of Pain and Symptom Management, 19*, 240-248.

Reuben, D., Herr, K., Pacala, J., Pollack, B., Potter, J., & Semla, T. (2005). *Geriatrics at your fingertips* (2005 ed.). Belle Meade, NJ: Excerpta Medica, Inc.

Richards, R., Nepomuceno, C., Riles, M., & Suer, A. (1982). Assessing pain behavior: The UAB Pain Behavior Scale. *Pain, 14*, 393-398.

Scherder, E., Oosterman, J., Swaab, D., Herr, K., Ooms, M., Ribbe, M., et al. (2005). Recent developments in pain in dementia. *British Medical Journal, 330,* 461-464.

Scherder, E. J. A., Slaets, J., Deijen, J. B., Gorter, Y., Ooms, M. E., Ribbe, M., et al. (2003). Pain assessment in patients with possible vascular dementia. *Psychiatry, 66*(2), 133-145.

Schuler, M., Njoo, N., Hestermann, M., Oster, P., & Hauer, K. (2004). Acute and chronic pain in geriatrics: Clinical characteristics of pain and the influence of cognition. *Pain Medicine, 5*(3), 253-262.

Shega, J. W., Hougham, G. W., Stocking, C. B., Cox-Hayley, D., & Sachs, G. A. (2004). Pain in community-dwelling persons with dementia: Frequency, intensity, and congruence between patient and caregiver report. *Journal of Pain and Symptom Management, 28*(6), 585-592.

Snow, A. L., Weber, J. B., O'Malley, K. J., Cody, M., Beck, C., Bruera, E., et al. (2004). NOPPAIN: A nursing assistant-administered pain assessment instrument for use in dementia. *Dementia and Geriatric Cognitive Disorders, 17*(3), 240-246.

Taylor, L. J., & Herr, K. (2003). Pain intensity assessment: A comparison of selected pain intensity scales for use in cognitively intact and cognitively impaired African-American older adults. *Pain Management Nursing, 4*(2), 87-95.

Taylor, L. J., Harris, J., Epps, C., & Herr, K. (2005). Psychometric evaluation of selected pain intensity scales for use in cognitively impaired and cognitively intact older adults. *Rehabilitation Nursing, 30*(2), 55-61.

Teno, J., Weitzen, S., Wetle, T., & Mor, V. (2001). Persistent pain in nursing home residents. *Journal of the American Medical Association, 285*(16), 2081.

Teno, J. M., Kabunoto, G., Wetle, T., Roy, J., & Mor, V. (2004). Daily pain that was excruciating at some time in the previous week: Prevalence, characteristics, and outcomes in nursing home residents. *Journal of the American Geriatrics Society, 52*(5), 762-767.

Warden, V., Hurley, A. C., & Volicer, L. (2003). Development and psychometric evaluation of the pain assessment in advanced dementia (PAINAD) scale. *Journal of the American Medical Directors Association,* Jan./Feb., 9-15.

Weiner, D., & Herr, K. (2002). Comprehensive interdisciplinary assessment and treatment planning: An integrative overview. In D. Weiner, K. Herr, & T. Rudy (Eds.), *Persistent pain in older adults: An interdisciplinary guide for treatment* (pp. 18-57). New York: Springer Publishing Company.

Weiner, D., Herr, K., & Rudy, T. (Eds.). (2002). *Persistent pain in older adults: An interdisciplinary guide for treatment.* New York: Springer Publishing Company.

Weiner, D., Peterson, B., & Keefe, F. (1999). Chronic pain-associated behaviors in the nursing home: Resident versus caregiver perceptions. *Pain, 80,* 577-588.

Weiner, D., Peterson, B., Ladd, K., McConnell, E., & Keefe, F. (1999). Pain in nursing home residents: An exploration of prevalence, staff perspectives, and practical aspects of measurement. *Clinical Journal of Pain, 15,* 92-101.

Weiner, D., Pieper, C., McConnell, E., Martinez, S., & Keefe, F. (1996). Pain measurement in elders with chronic low back pain: Traditional and alternative approaches. *Pain, 67,* 461-467.

Won, A., Lapane, K., Gambassi, G., Bernabei, R., Mor, V., & Lipsitz, L. A. (1999). Correlates and management of nonmalignant pain in the nursing home. *Journal of the American Geriatrics Society, 47,* 936-942.

Won, A. B., Lapane, K. L., Vallow, S., Schein, J., Morris, J. N., & Lipsitz, L. A. (2004). Persistent nonmalignant pain and analgesic prescribing patterns in elderly nursing home residents. *Journal of the American Geriatrics Society, 52*(6), 867-874.

Yeager, K. A., Miaskowski, C., Dibble, S. L., & Wallhagen, M. (1995). Differences in pain knowledge and experience between oncology outpatients and their caregivers. *Oncology Nursing Forum, 22,* 1235-1241.

ASSESSING PAIN IN A PERSON WITH DEMENTIA

My mother is dying of Parkinson's disease and also has dementia. Recently she has been making strange sounds and, at the same time, blinking her eyes rapidly. This does not occur all the time, but these actions seem to be increasing in frequency. Are her actions simply part of her conditions, or could they be a signal of pain?

■   ■   ■

It is important for you to consider yourself part of the team caring for your mom. Your observations can assist health professionals assess and treat her effectively. You are correct to consider that your mother's actions may be a sign that she is in pain. I am assuming that your mother can no longer communicate with you in traditional ways and therefore cannot effectively describe her pain.

Share your observations with the doctors and nurses who are treating your mother. They (and you) may want to make further observations. Are her actions at a particular time of day, such as after meals, medications, or other events? What other activities or procedures are going on when you observe such behaviors? In short, can you see anything that might create a change and account for your mother's new behavior?

The next step would be for the medical team to review your mother's medical history, considering new conditions, progression of her disease, and other chronic illnesses she is experiencing. Often, an analgesic trial can help sort things out. Here pain medication is administered or increased to see if it affects the observed behaviors. If, for example, the dosage of your mother's analgesic medication is increased and her sounds and blinking decrease or end, this would be a good indication that pain was the factor behind her actions.

It is often difficult to assess pain in someone with dementia. That is why it is important that family members like you become actively involved by sharing your observations and by advocating for your mother.

■ CHAPTER 7 ■

End-of-Life Pain Management in Children and Adolescents

By Rebecca Selove, Dianne Cochran, and Ira Todd Cohen

INTRODUCTION

As health care professionals, we are just beginning to acknowledge the fact that life sometimes ends during childhood. This sad but undeniable truth was once integrated into the human experience, but with advances in nutrition, sanitation, and technology, modern society has distanced itself from this painful reality. Unlike palliative care in adults, the treatment of pain and other forms of suffering associated with life-threatening disorders in children has only just begun to be explored (Field & Berman, 2003). Family and staff are understandably reluctant to give up hope and frequently delay palliative interventions until the last days or even hours of life. The growing number of professionals dedicated to improving the quality of life of dying children must address and manage their own "strong emotional and professional tensions, psychologic and emotional responses, and religious, spiritual and philosophical reactions" (Perilongo et al., 2001, p. 59) to the impending death of a young person in order to provide high-quality, integrated care.

Effective pain management in this arena requires that pediatric health care providers take into account the multitude of physiologic and psychological changes that occur from infancy through adolescence, including changes in relationships with parents (Thompson & Varni, 1986; Twycross, 1998). Physiologically and pharmacologically, neonates and infants exhibit renal, hepatic, and blood-brain barrier compromise. With maturation, these functions slowly approach those of healthy adults, but special considerations are still required when selecting analgesics, doses, and modalities during childhood. Assessing a specific child's conceptualization of what causes and eases pain, understanding of time, ability to implement behavioral and cognitive strategies for coping with pain, and psychosocial issues associated with this child's stage of development provides caregivers with crucial information for addressing the physical and emotional issues a child and his or her family face as death nears.

In addition, in order to provide adequate care for children and adolescents, the role and emotional needs of their family members must be considered. The child's comfort can be enhanced when parents experience support and guidance for their own grieving process and for involving siblings in age-appropriate ways. Parents can then more effectively contribute to the plan for treating their child's pain, have more confidence in its effectiveness, and sincerely reassure their child that pain relief is on the way.

Chaffee (2001) described numerous barriers to effective pain management for children at the end of life, including factors associated with the knowledge, awareness, and emotions of health care providers, parents, and patients, as well as factors associated with the physiology of pain and with analgesic and opioid treatments. She advocated a "multimodal approach" (p. 381) with provision of pharmacologic as well as cognitive, behavioral, and physical interventions. In this chapter we follow this multimodal approach, using patient age ranges to frame discussion of relevant physiological and psychosocial issues and interventions.

NEONATES AND INFANTS

*Full acknowledgment of neonatal dignity and personhood
is a prerequisite for an effective treatment of
neonatal pain.* (Bellieni, 2005, p. 5)

Death in children under 1 year of age, excluding perinatal mortality, most commonly arises from congenital malformations and complications of premature birth (Leuthner, 2004; Pierucci, Kirby, & Leuthner, 2001). Both of these broad categories of disorders frequently require multiple surgical interventions and ongoing invasive procedures. In addition, prolonged periods of mechanical ventilation and repeated diagnostic tests subject these infants to persistent and, at times, extreme pain. Many of these infants, if they are not severely compromised, may survive for weeks, even months, experiencing all the discomforts and complications of an intensive care setting (Carter, 2005).

An infant's ability to sense and respond to painful or noxious stimuli has been well documented over the past two decades (Fitzgerald, 2005; Wolf, 1999). By 20 weeks gestation, cerebral, spinal, and peripheral neurodevelopment has achieved thalamic-neocortical arborization, spinothalamic interconnections, and cutaneous sensory neuronal density equivalent to that found in adults. Myelination and inhibitory pathways are still developing after birth, allowing for slow but sustained nociception. In term infants, opioid binding sites are found in greater number in the cerebellum than in adults, and measured brain activity is maximal in sensory areas.

Behavioral and physiological responses of infants strongly suggest that their response to pain is much more than reflexive. Reproducible facial expressions such as forehead bulging, eye closing, and nasolabial furrowing have been observed in both adults and infants with a variety of pain modalities. In the neonate, heart rate, blood pressure, intracranial pressure, and sweating all increase with painful stimuli. Persistent hypersensitivity has been documented in infants who have experienced heel sticks and circumcision without analgesia, demonstrated by increased withdrawal response, prolonged crying, sleep disturbance, and poor feeding. Older infants might also exhibit physical resistance by pushing the stimulus away after it is applied, attempting to withdraw, opening eyes with a look of anger, and crying loudly.

Providing effective pain management at the end of life starts with a complete pain assessment. Various observational pain assessment scales such as the Neonatal Infant Pain Scale (NIPS) (Lawrence et al., 1993) or CRIES (Crying, Requires increased oxygen, Increased vital signs, Expression, Sleeplessness) (Krechel & Bildner, 1995) provide professionals with standardized tools for evaluating and documenting pain. These instruments use the signs and symptoms described in the previous paragraph. Health professionals can maximize pain management through regular and frequent assessments, intervention planning, and administration of pharmacological treatments. It is imperative that clinicians provide ongoing family education regarding expected disease trajectory-related symptoms of pain and the necessity to report symptoms or changes as they are observed.

Compassionate care and symptom management by health professionals can help patients and their families transition from a curative model to a focus on palliative support. We best serve families by acknowledging our limited ability to cure while assuring them that much can be done to ensure their child's comfort at the end of life. While striving to manage symptoms, clinicians are challenged to provide intimate, quiet time for the families to develop memories with their infant and to cope with the impending loss.

The immature physiology of infants often limits practitioners' choice and dosing of analgesic medications. Comparatively insufficient renal and hepatic function decreases clearance and metabolism of most medications. Lower serum protein levels decrease binding of medications and their metabolites. These factors increase drug serum levels in infants, necessitating lower doses, longer dosing intervals, and, in some cases, total avoidance. In addition, the incomplete formation of the blood-brain barrier allows more rapid and greater amounts of hydrophilic medication, such as morphine, to enter the central nervous system (Nandi & Fitzgerald, 2005). Studies of analgesics in the infant population are limited. Medication use often falls outside the Food and Drug Administration's labeling recommendations.

Establishing steady-state analgesic serum levels, which minimize the risk of undertreatment, side effects, and drug toxicity, is ideal for all patients but is essential in infants. Around-the-clock dosing of oral and rectal medications and continuous infusions of intravenous drugs are strongly recommended (Table 1). Morphine sulfate and fentanyl are often the opioids of choice, because data are available for this age group. Tolerance to fentanyl occurs within two to three days, making morphine a superior option (Suresh & Anand, 2001; Taddio, & Katz, 2004). Methadone, after optimal opioid dosing is determined, offers the advantages of its long half-life, availability in oral form, and antagonism of the NMDA receptors (Chana & Anand, 2001). Experience is limited for the use of adjunct medications in infants. Beh and Kearns (2001) report on the efficacy of gabapentin in infants with chronic pain.

Regional anesthetic techniques should also be considered in this age group (Table 2). Epidural infusions via indwelling catheters can achieve remarkable relief of somatic, visceral, and neuropathic pain (Galloway & Yaster, 2000). In infants, many local anesthetics have narrow safety profiles in which therapeutic doses often approach levels of toxicity. Ropivacaine has decreased cardio-depression, arrhythmogenicity, and serum free-fraction compared with bupivacaine, making its use relatively safer in this age group. If appropriate, peripheral nerve blocks can also be considered for diagnostic purposes and limited treatment.

Because infants are unable to verbalize the location and nature of their pain, caregivers rely on other sources of information to formulate their ideas about the cause of a baby's distress. Parents' beliefs and emotions related to their child, as well as the family's history, configuration, and dynamics, can all affect the parents' interpretation of a baby's fussiness, withdrawal, or lethargy. Understanding the parents' perspective is crucial, because treatment team members use parents' observations and perceptions in making decisions about pain management and because they aim to provide reassuring feedback to family members regarding the baby's behavior and mood. Asking family members about their observations demonstrates a welcoming interest in their involvement in the child's care.

Psychosocial interventions that focus on parents and other caregivers complement medical and pharmacological interventions for reducing pain and distress in neonates and infants. Parents and other familiar people

TABLE 1. PEDIATRIC ANALGESIC MEDICATIONS FOR END-OF-LIFE PAIN

Medication	Route	Dose/kg (q 4-6h)	Nota Bene
Nonopioids			
Acetaminophen	Oral	10-15 mg/kg	Infant: 5-8 mg/kg q 6h
Acetaminophen	Rectal	Load: 30-40 mg/kg →20 mg/kg q 6h	(−) Immunodeficiency
Ibuprofen	Oral	10 mg/kg/	(−) Coagulopathy, Oncology patients
Ketoralac	Oral, IV	Load: 0.5 mg/kg →0.25 mg/kg q 6h	(−) Renal insufficiency; use limited to 5 days
Tramadol	Oral	1-2 mg/kg	(−) Use of Selective serotonin reuptake inhibitor
Opioids			
Codeine	Oral	0.5-1 mg/kg	Ineffective for 20% of patients
Oxycodone	Oral	0.05-0.15 mg/kg	
Morphine sulfate	Oral	0.2-0.5 mg/kg	Morphine sulfate immediate release
Morphine sulfate	IV, SQ	0.1 mg/kg	
Morphine sulfate	IV Infusion	0.02 mg/kg/h	Patient Controlled Analgesia (PCA) (self or nurse-assist)
Hydromorphone	Oral	0.03-0.08 mg/kg	
Hydromorphone	IV	0.015 mg/kg	
Hydromorphone	IV Infusion	0.003 mg/kg/h	PCA (self or nurse-assist)
Methadone	Oral, IV	0.1 mg/kg q 6h	↑ Half-life with exposure
Fentanyl	IV Infusion	1 microgram/kg/h	Rapid onset of tolerance
— Patch	Transdermal	1 microgram/kg q 3d	(−) Opioid naïve patient
— Oralet	Transmucosal	5-15 micrograms/kg	(−) Infants < 15 kg
Adjuncts			
Gabapentin	Oral	5 mg/kg; Day 1 q hs Day 2 q 12h, Day 3 q 8h	(+) Neuropathic pain; advance gradually
Nortriptyline	Oral	0.1-0.5 mg q hs	(+) Neuropathic pain; advance gradually
Mexiletine	Oral	2-3 mg/kg q 6-8h; increase very slowly	(+) Neuropathic pain; (−) Seizure, cardiac
Lorazepam	Oral, IV	0.02-0.1 mg/kg q 8h	(+) Spasm, anxiety
Ketamine	IV Infusion	0.1-0.5 mg/kg/h	↓ Opioid tolerance
Lidocaine	IV Infusion	2-5 mg/kg/h	Monitor for toxicity
Clonidine	Oral	2-4 micrograms/kg	(+) Neuro/visceral pain
— Patch	Transdermal	0.1-0.2 mg/kg q 7d	(−) Hypotension

All doses q 4-6h unless otherwise noted; IV = intravenous; ↑ = increase; ↓ = decrease; SQ = subcutaneous; q = every; h = hour; d = day; → = then; hs = hour of sleep; (−) = contraindicated; (+) = therapeutic

The information in the tables is drawn from the multiple sources cited in the text.

TABLE 2. PEDIATRIC REGIONAL ANALGESIA FOR END-OF-LIFE PAIN

Technique	Rate/Dose	Risk/Benefit	Possible Side Effects
Epidural	0.2-0.4 ml/kg/h	Infection, hematoma, urinary retention, weakness	
▪ Morphine	20 micrograms/ml	Rostral spread	Sedation, ↓ RR, pruritis
▪ Hydromorphone	10 micrograms/ml	Rostral spread	Sedation, ↓ RR, pruritis
▪ Fentanyl	1-2 micrograms/ml	Systemic absorption	Pruritis, sedation, ↓ RR
▪ Clonidine	0.1 microgram/ml	↓ Blood pressure	Sedation, hypotension
▪ Bupivacaine	0.1%	Toxic > 0.4 ml/kg/h	Tinnitus, disinhibition,
▪ Ropivacaine	0.1%	Safer toxicity profile	Seizures, dysrhythmias
Nerve Block		**Administration**	
▪ Bupivacaine	0.5 ml/kg (0.25%)	Single dose only	See above
▪ Lidocaine	0.5 ml/kg (0.1%)	Single dose only	See above
▪ Ropivacaine	0.1-0.3 ml/kg/h (0.2%)	Catheter for infusion	Infection, signs of toxicity
▪ Levobupivacaine	0.1 ml/kg/h (0.25%)	Catheter for infusion	Infection, signs of toxicity
▪ Neurolysis	Alcohol or phenol	Ablation of nerve	Loss of function
Cutaneous		**Penetration**	
▪ EMLA®	Lidocaine/prilocaine (2.5%)	After 90 min, 5 mm	Methemoglobin, blenching
▪ ELA-max® [no "M"]	Liposomal Lidocaine 4 %	After 30 min, 5 mm	Lidocaine toxicity
▪ Lidoderm® Patch	12 hours on/off (5%)	Dermal analgesia	Only approved for PHN

RR = respiratory rate; EMLA = eutectic mixture of lidocaine and prilocaine; PHN = post-herpetic neuralgia

The information in the tables is drawn from the multiple sources cited in the text.

are usually most able to comfort infants and can provide blankets or favorite toys from home for those times when they can't be present. They may recommend certain positions that have helped comfort their baby in the past or provide music or recordings of themselves and other relatives talking or singing.

In many medical settings, chaplains, psychologists, and social workers provide compassionate listening so that family members experience being understood in their worry and grief. Sometimes these members of the team facilitate communication between various health care professionals and the parents, which can reduce parents' anxiety so that they can focus more effectively on soothing their child.

TODDLERS

> *A person's a person no matter how small.*
> (Geisel, 1954 [aka Dr. Seuss])

Beyond the first year of life, the most common cause of death during childhood is unintentional and inflicted trauma. In 2002, in the United States, trauma accounted for deaths in 42.5% of 1- to 4-year-old children (Anderson & Smith, 2005), with traumatic brain injury (TBI) accounting for the largest percentage of deaths. In the 1990s, the death rate due to TBI was 6.7 per 100,000 for children under 4 years (Adekoya, Thurman, White, & Webb, 2002). These children often require intracranial and intravascular monitoring, ventilatory support, and numerous diagnostic procedures. Cardiovascular function in these otherwise healthy trauma victims will often remain stable until brain death is confirmed and supportive measures are withdrawn.

Assessing toddlers with a terminal illness can and should involve creativity from the practitioner. Sick toddlers still find pleasure and comfort in play activities, and games like "Simon Says"; drawing; stacking blocks; singing; and playing with stuffed animals, dolls, or puppets can provide a window into the individual patient while minimizing disruption of family time. Participating in a toddler's play allows the professional to assess important aspects of a child's pain. Is it harder for a child to move from Mom's lap to color at a play table? Is the child no longer able to ride

FIGURE 1. WONG-BAKER FACES PAIN RATING SCALE

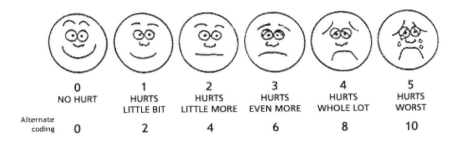

From Wong's *Essential Pediatric Nursing* (7th ed.) (p. 1259), by M. J. Hockenberry, D. Wilson, & M. L. Winkerstein, 2005, St. Louis, MO: Mosby. Copyright, Mosby. Used with permission.

a tricycle up and down the hallway? Does it seem that a child cannot find a comfortable position on Dad's lap because of pain? Parents can help with pain assessment by telling the professional what words are familiar to the child for describing pain.

Most toddlers can report general information such as "it hurts a lot," point to the part on their body that hurts, and use pain tools such as the FLACC (Face, Legs, Activity, Cry, and Consolable) scale (Merkel, Voepel-Lewis, Shayevitz, & Malviya, 1997) or the Wong-Baker FACES pain rating scale (Figure 1). However, they have not yet developed the ability to describe pain in detail, use qualitative descriptors, or accurately localize symptoms.

Toddlers and preschoolers might deny pain for fear of having another painful exam or to avoid taking bad-tasting medication. Children between the ages of 1 and 4 years might exhibit increased intensity of pain with periods of hysterical crying or rigid body posture. Insight into pain locations can be gained by observing toddlers patting the body parts that hurt. They may frown or grimace during physical exams, withdraw from beloved activities, or become disinterested in their surroundings as part of their response to increased pain.

Pain can provoke intense emotional distress in toddlers. Children ages 2 through 7 generally do not understand pain as caused by illness or efforts to treat them; instead, they are prone to experiencing guilt for the wrongs they think required the punishment of illness and medical procedures. They may also express anger at parents, nurses, and other medical staff for allowing or causing pain to occur. Verbal expressions of pain by children in this age range and older can reflect physical as well as emotional distress, such as fear of separation from their parents. Emotional pain is sometimes more difficult to describe, even for older children and adolescents.

Furthermore, a myriad of situational factors that are not consistently associated with age, gender, or medical condition modify the experience and expression of pain in children and adolescents (McGrath & Hillier, 2003). These factors may include behavior of staff that provide care, parents' approach to coping with their child's illness, parents' attitudes and behavior in relation to staff, and the impact of the child's illness on the family. In assessing the pain of a toddler, the practitioner needs to consider the situational and relational dimensions of the child's perspective in addition to the illness and the analgesic pharmacological processes.

In the toddler age group there are more options for pain intervention than with infants, but limiting factors include a child's level of cognitive development, inability to swallow pills, and body weight too low for standardized medications and delivery systems. Around-the-clock use of oral elixirs and continuous infusions are indicated for these patients, who are unlikely to advocate for themselves (Hain, Miser, Devins, & Wallace, 2005). The presence of concrete cognitive function and magical thinking makes toddlers poor candidates for patient-controlled analgesia (PCA). Nurse-assist PCA has achieved successful pain management by increasing incremental dosing and interval times (Galloway & Yaster, 2000). As with infants, regional anesthetic techniques can offer alternative approaches (Dadure & Capdevila, 2005; Suresh & Wheeler, 2002).

Long-acting, sustained-released oral opioids depend on embedding the active agent in slowly digested matrixes. Crushing or compounding these medications is contraindicated. Capsules, which are typically formulated in doses too high for the weight of a toddler and are difficult to swallow, are not an option. Methadone, as a tablet or an elixir, offers the advantage of a long half-life that increases with exposure to the medica-tion. Dosing can be changed from every 6 hours to every 8 or 12 hours within days or weeks. Adjuncts such as gabapentin, lorazepam, and clonidine can be compounded as liquids (Table 1). Transdermal patches do not exist in dose sizes for these patients, who are typically less than 20 kilograms. Intravenous lidocaine infusion is a viable alternative in toddlers with neuropathic or intractable pain (Massey, Pedigo, Dunn, Grossman, & Russell, 2002).

Psychosocial interventions for toddlers and young children include reinforcing their cooperative behaviors with verbal praise and sticker charts. It is important to make explicit statements about the fact that illness is not a consequence of anything the child did and that adults regret that some treatments are painful and will take steps, such as using topical anesthetics, to reduce discomfort.

Health care providers can help prepare children for procedures, transitions from one place to another, and other aspects of care with simple but concrete explanations of what is planned and why. Child Life Specialists are trained in the use of medical toys and specially constructed dolls for giving children opportunities to see, ahead of time, a version of what they will experience later. In the context of play, children are sometimes able to express fears and anger, as well as to develop a sense of mastery that helps them be more relaxed, which is associated with lowered pain and distress. Family members and Child Life Specialists can also provide relaxing and distracting activities according to a child's interests, such as watching movies, drawing and coloring, or having stories read to him or her.

Attention to the contexts in which a child experiences pain may yield important information about situational factors that exacerbate distress. The presence or absence of family members, as well as the mood and activity of those present, can contribute to or alleviate stress to some degree. While it may not be immediately apparent, stressful events in the patient's room may make it more difficult for the child to relax or rest. Health care providers and psychosocial team members can model (and coach staff and family members in the use of) discretion regarding topics that are discussed in the child's presence, talking calmly and confidently about day-to-day and hour-to-hour plans, and validating the toddler's emotions.

CHILDREN

The aims of pediatric palliative care should [be] improving the quality of life, maintaining the dignity, and ameliorating the suffering of seriously ill or dying children in ways that are appropriate to their upbringing, culture, and community.
(Himelstein, Hilden, Boldt, & Weissman, 2004, p. 1752)

Neoplasms account for approximately 20% of deaths that occur in children between 5 and 12 years of age (Bradshaw, Hinds, Lensing, Gattuso, & Razzouk, 2004). Childhood cancers are the diseases typically considered when health care providers discuss pediatric palliative care. Pain and discomfort can originate directly from the disease or as a result of medical or surgical intervention. In this patient population, it is not uncommon to encounter all three categories of pain: somatic (bone, muscle, and mucosa), visceral (hollow and solid internal organs), and neuropathic (nerve impingement, injury, and amputation). In addition, these patients may experience numerous hospital admissions, clinic visits, and diagnostic procedures that further sensitize them to pain and other symptoms.

Children under age 10 may understand pain associated with trauma more easily than pain associated with disease, because they are operating at a more concrete cognitive level (Twycross, 1998). They may describe their pain in vague terms and may be better able to indicate the location of their pain by pointing to their own body, a drawn outline of a body, or a simple doll rather than describing it in words. Children 10 to 12 years old can usually verbalize where they hurt and what has provided relief in the past more precisely than younger children can. As they get older, children are more likely to associate pain with some kind of injury to their body, including illness and disease that has no external cause. They are also more able than toddlers to collaborate with caregivers in considering various interventions.

Children can be exquisitely sensitive to their caregivers' reactions and moods, and their reports of pain may be affected by their efforts to cope with family dynamics. For instance, a child may deny pain even while grimacing if the parent seems anxious about pain as a sign that the child's condition is deteriorating. A child may complain of pain and ask for more comfort measures as a way of distracting parents who are perceived to be arguing with each other or are talking about other stresses in their lives. This is not to say that the child is not in pain; rather, because there are physiological repercussions of emotional stress, we could say that the child is attempting to change an interpersonal dynamic in an effort to reduce his or her pain.

In the context of a trusted relationship, children are more likely to describe their pain and express their feelings openly. In her ground-breaking book *The Private Worlds of Dying Children,* Bluebond-Langner (1978) wrote,

> [C]hildren…were faced with constant conflict. Even the decision to reveal one's awareness directly was fraught with questions of to whom and when. There were always risks involved. If the children used a distancing strategy that other people did not like, or if they attempted to reveal their knowledge and others did not accept it, they might be abandoned. (p. 228)

Respectful attention and responses to a child's activities and words can foster trust in a care provider.

School-age children can be more actively involved in their own pain assessment than younger ones. Children who have been receiving medical care for ongoing health problems are usually familiar with standard pain tools such as FACES or visual analog pain scales. It is common for children in this age group to seek information as to why the pain is increasing. Being honest and involving the children and their families in determining the plan of care can lead to significantly better symptom management.

Children may have multiple pain sites and types of pain. It is important to address their concerns and those of family members about the different pain locations and to continually reassess their pain after implementing treatment. Children should not be expected to make major decisions, but it is important to provide ways for them to participate in their care.

Allowing school-age children to participate in their care includes letting them use PCA and patient-controlled epidural anesthesia (PCEA). Because they are larger than toddlers and may need prolonged exposure to opioids, it may be possible to implement transdermal, transmucosal

(Susman, 2005), or intraspinal (Saroyan, Schechter, Tresgallo, & Granowetter, 2005) delivery systems in these patients. Ideally, these modes of delivery should be reserved for patients who are unable to take oral medications or whose pain is poorly controlled by them. In all age groups, prolonged exposure to opioids will result in the need for increasing doses. To avoid this escalation, ultralow (nonanesthetic or sedative) dose infusions of ketamine can be effective in preventing the development of opioid tolerance (Subramaniam, Subramaniam, & Steinbrook, 2004).

Adjuncts available in tablet form—such as gabapentin, nortriptyline, and mexiletine—should be considered for patients with neuropathic pain. Mexiletine is an oral antiarrhythmic that has a lidocaine-like effect in treating neuropathic and intractable pain (Galloway & Yaster, 2000). The medications and techniques discussed for infants and toddlers can also be used in the school-age child, especially when psychological regression and medical debilitation interfere with mental and psychomotor function. It is important to recognize that doses of medications must be individualized to the intensity of pain being experienced and specific to the age-determined physiology, and to determine the correct delivery system for a particular child and that child's family.

Steroids, chemotherapy, radiation, and debulking procedures, which reduce tumors impinging on anatomical structures or nerves, may reduce pain in cancer patients. Regional techniques and nerve blocks can also be effective. If nerve blocks are successful, neurolysis should be offered, with the understanding that loss of associated function will be permanent (Table 2).

Children in the early elementary school years and younger may not be reassured if they are told that some unpleasant procedure or oral medication will make them feel better; at their level of cognitive development, the parent's kiss and the bandage have more comforting power. Children this age and older may be soothed by hearing their parents reminisce about their lives and review family photographs. Witnessing the meaningfulness of their lives through the voices and memories of their parents can be reassuring to children facing the end of life.

Development of sleeping difficulties is not unusual in children nearing the end of life. They may become anxious about being alone at night, fearful that they will die while they are asleep, or worried that their parents will be unable to cope with their death. Preparing parents for the possibility of nighttime fears and helping them create a plan for supporting their child is another important part of care. Parents can use bedtime rituals such as reading or telling stories, sharing relaxing images, and focusing on slow, rhythmic breathing to model and support preparing the mind and body for rest. At all stages of a young person's life, a parent's physical contact can be of tremendous comfort. It may take the form of holding a hand, cuddling, or rubbing feet for younger children, and more elaborate massage techniques for older children and teenagers.

Most children in the later elementary years have developed cognitive abilities that allow additional behavioral interventions to be added to those previously described. Many children can help plan for distracting activities, practice relaxation techniques such as focusing on their breath and using imagery, and talk about the relationships among factors such as worrisome thoughts, difficulty sleeping, and increased pain and distress. Some children like to be asked questions to elicit a detailed description of what is in a favorite room at home or what they did on their Make-A-Wish trip. Parents can enhance the effectiveness of relaxation techniques by integrating them into the times when their child is relatively comfortable and better able to concentrate on the activity.

Children and adolescents may need help expressing their thoughts, desires, and grief for the dreams they are unable to fulfill. One should consider what goals a child may want to achieve as his or her life is ending. Some young people who feel secure with their caregivers may ask questions about what it will be like to die and what their families will do after their death. A counselor from the family's faith community or a hospital chaplain who has been trained to work with young people may help them express their preferences for their own memorial services and disposition of their personal belongings.

When home hospice is being discussed as an option, children and families might indicate that they fear giving up the "safety" of the hospital and established relationships with professional caregivers. Parents may be anxious about living in the house after their child has died there. It can be helpful to have hospice staff meet the child and family in the hospital to answer questions and begin the process of becoming familiar to the family.

ADOLESCENTS

> *Parties shall assure to the child who is capable of forming his or her own views the right to express those views freely in all manners affecting the child, the views of the child being given due weight in accordance with the age and maturity of the child.* (United Nations, 1989)

Teenage patients may experience death secondary to trauma, neoplasms, and other less frequent causes. Genetic and acquired disorders such as cystic fibrosis, sickle cell anemia, and AIDS may become lethal in the second decade of life. Pain may arise from chronic conditions such as pancreatitis, sinusitis, and aseptic necrosis. Although physiologically similar to adults, these patients require special consideration, as they are at a time of life during which growth, puberty, and independence are the norm (Freyer, 2004).

Teens often want to be involved with their care plan and pain assessment, and to be shown respect by having their questions answered truthfully. They can verbalize their level of pain using the visual analog scale, the numeric scale, and even the FACES pain scale. A teenager can be asked to describe the intensity, quality, and any patterns of pain he or she has noticed, such as aggravating factors and anything that has helped to alleviate pain. A Pain Diary can be useful for some adolescents as a means for keeping track of changes in pain in relation to their activities, mood, and pain interventions. Asking what the adolescent thinks the pain means and how it affects activities of daily living can yield key information.

Adolescents can be supported with explicit messages to the effect that they are an important part of the team and their thoughts and ideas will be integrated into the care plan. Sensitivity regarding the pace at which they process information and find words to express themselves increases their comfort with the assessment process, as does respect for their physical privacy.

While in physical appearance, vocabulary, and sometimes demeanor an adolescent may appear to be grown up, we serve them better if we remember the aspects of cognitive and emotional development that distinguish them from adults. Furthermore, considering the social and medical history of the individual adolescent patient will allow us to be more in sync with what that person needs to be more comfortable. The perspective of a child with a chronic illness, many years of treatment, or an earlier history of treatment followed by remission and then relapse will be quite different from that of a child with a recent or sudden onset of a life-threatening condition.

One of the best known characteristics of adolescents is thinking that they are old enough to make many significant decisions for themselves and wanting to be seen as competent, while at the same time often feeling anxious about making mistakes and knowing that they aren't able to comprehend everything that is needed for decision making in complex situations. Ideally, health caregivers aim to honor both sides of the seesaw: the adolescent's wish to be consulted and the wish to involve supportive adults who provide input and reassurance. It can be very important to engage the adolescent in the process of assessing and treating pain, while recognizing that parents' input, judiciously timed and phrased, can enhance a teenager's sense of control in treatment decisions. Health care professionals can model respectful inclusion of the teenager's attitudes and feelings during conversations with parents. This is a way of proactively addressing the teenager's yearning to be respected as an autonomous individual.

Some adolescents will appreciate education about the team's approach to pain management, perhaps with ABCDE (Assess, Believe, Choose, Deliver, Empower) and PQRST (Precipitating Factors, Quality, Radiation, Severity/site, Time). Adolescents may need clarification of the differences among drug tolerance, physical dependence, and addiction. One should address and dispel the myth that the strongest medications are always saved for last.

Journaling can be useful for some adolescents as a means for reflecting on other aspects of their experience and life. Their goals and priorities may change as they grapple with the realization that their life is ending, and writing about their thoughts can sometimes help them clarify what they want to communicate to others. The clinician's goal is to prevent the adolescent from experiencing unnecessary or uncontrolled pain throughout this difficult journey.

Adolescents facing the end of life may obtain significant relief from distress by being able to create tangible expressions of their values, feelings, and memories. Paintings and sculpture, poetry, musical compositions and recordings, scrapbooks, and other crafts can be ways for teenagers to "leave a legacy" (Hain, Weinstein, Oleske, Orloff, & Cohen, 2004, p. 192). One teenager posted a testimonial to his faith on a Web page that his parents shared proudly; he said it gave him great comfort to think that he might help others he would never meet in person. Such activities can help a teenager relax during the creative period as well as provide spiritual comfort because the teenager is able to experience a sense of his or her impact on the world as continuing even after death.

Regression, depression, and "normal" adolescent opposition can interfere with a teenage patient's participation in pain management. Both assessment and treatment may be disrupted. By being patient and respectfully listening to an adolescent complain or argue, the practitioner may be able to convey acceptance of a range of thoughts and emotions, and help the young person see the practitioner as an ally.

Although the medications and modalities used in adults are available to this age group, they may not be appropriate or acceptable to individual patients. The untoward effects of therapy may be more intrusive or uncomfortable than the symptoms it is designed to address. For example, an additional intravenous line, epidural catheters, or disturbance of a preferred routine may be unwelcome.

Prevention or reduction of medication side effects is important in all age groups. Pruritis, nausea, vomiting, constipation, lethargy, and altered sensorium can sometimes be as distressing as pain to patients and their families. Antihistamines, serotonin antagonists, laxatives, stimulants, and altering medication schedules should all be considered. Wolfe and colleagues (2000) report that although pain was the number one concern of the end-of-life patients and their families, oversedation was also highly ranked and was not adequately recognized or addressed by the health care team. The children and their parents wanted wakeful periods so that life could be lived before death arrived.

CONCLUSION

The multimodal approach to providing end-of-life pain management for children and adolescents includes integrating pharmacological and psychosocial care with consideration of each patient's physical, cognitive, emotional, and spiritual level of development. Furthermore, quality care depends on clear and ongoing communication among members of the medical team and with the patient and his or her family. It may be helpful to identify a member of the team who will take responsibility for coordinating and monitoring each participant's satisfaction with the flow and timeliness of information.

A final and important aspect of end-of-life pain management is attention to the emotional well-being of the staff that provide care. Perilongo et al. (2001) and others (e.g., Burns, Mitchell, Griffith, & Truog, 2001; Sahler, Frager, Levetown, Cohn, & Lipson, 2000) have noted that being with young people (and with their families) at the end of their lives requires an enormous amount of giving from staff. Over time, health care professionals can become intimately familiar with and supportive of many patients, and develop meaningful relationships with them and their families. Health care providers witness intense love, fear, despair, and grief, and over the course of their professional lives they may experience many losses. In order for them to come to work each day ready to be caring, they must develop personal coping skills and strategies, which include engaging in mutually supportive relationships with colleagues. Each system within which end-of-life care is provided can establish "an array of highly visible and readily available options" (Dixon, Vodde, Freeman, Higdon, & Mathieson, 2005) that fit the dynamics of the caregivers and the pace of care, so that caregivers will not have to search out a time and place to talk about someone who is dying or has died. By creating "debriefing" (Serwint, 2004) or memory-sharing opportunities, staff can design a supportive program that fits the unique character of their particular group. In this way they can enhance the quality of their work together, which will translate into better care for patients and their families. ■

Rebecca Selove, PhD, MPH is the Clinical Psychologist for the Department of Hematology/Oncology at Children's National Medical Center in Washington, DC. She received her graduate training at George Peabody College of Vanderbilt University and the Child Study Center at Yale University. She has worked with children and families in other hospitals as well as in public schools and community mental health centers. Her research interests include evaluation of the impact of psychosocial services for children with cancer and sickle cell disease and their families, as well as quality of life for long-term survivors of pediatric cancers.

Dianne Cochran, BSRN, received her Bachelor of Science of Nursing from West Virginia Wesleyan College. She has specialized in pediatrics for 22 years and maintained her certification of pediatrics nurse since 1995. Dianne has spent her clinical years at Children's National Medical Center Burn Intensive Care Unit/Burn step-down for 5 years, 11 years in Post Anesthesia Care and the past 6 years with the Anesthesia Pain Service. She is actively involved with Pain PI, Sickle Cell Committee, and the PANDA (Pediatric Advanced Needs Assessment and Care team) Committee.

Ira Todd Cohen, MD, is an Associate Professor of Anesthesiology and Pediatrics. He completed his residency in Pediatrics at the Albert Einstein Affiliate Hospitals and in Anesthesiology at the New York University Medical Center. He received further training during his fellowship in Pediatric Anesthesiology at Children's National Medical Center (CNMC) and in pain management at the Pittsburgh Pain Evaluation Treatment Institute. Dr. Cohen is an active member of Acute Pain Team and a founding member of the Palliative and End-of-Life Care Committee at CNMC.

REFERENCES

Adekoya, N., Thurman, D. J., White, D. D., & Webb, K. (2002). Surveillance for traumatic brain injury deaths-United States, 1989-1998. *Morbidity and Mortality Weekly Report, 51*, 1-14.

Anderson, R. N., & Smith, B. L. (2005). Deaths: Leading causes for 2002. *National Vital Statistics Report, 53*, 1-89.

Beh, M. O., & Kearns, G. L. (2001). Treatment of pain with gabapentin in a neonate. *Pediatrics, 108*, 482-484.

Bellieni, C. (2005). Pain definitions revised: Newborns not only feel pain, they also suffer. *Medical Ethics, Ethics Medical, 21*, 5-9.

Bluebond-Langner, M. (1978). *The private lives of dying children.* Princeton, NJ: Princeton University Press.

Bradshaw, G., Hinds, P. S., Lensing, S., Gattuso, J. S., & Razzouk, B. I. (2004). Cancer-related deaths in children and adolescents. *Journal of Palliative Medicine, 8*, 86–95.

Burns, J. P., Mitchell, C., Griffith, J. L., & Truog, R. D. (2001). End-of-life care in the pediatric intensive care unit: Attitudes and practices of pediatric critical care physicians and nurses. *Critical Care Medicine, 29*(3), 658-664.

Carter, B. S. (2005). Providing palliative care for newborns. *Pediatric Annals, 33*, 770–777.

Chaffee, S. (2001). Pediatric palliative care. *Primary Care Clinics in Office Practice, 28*, 365–390.

Chana, S. K., & Anand, K. J. (2001). Can we use methadone for analgesia in neonates? *Archives of Disease in Childhood, 85*, 79-81.

Dadure, C., & Capdevila, X. (2005). Continuous peripheral nerve blocks in children. *Clinical Anaesthesiology, 19*, 309-321.

Dixon, D., Vodde, R., Freeman, M., Higdon, T., & Mathieson, S. G. (2005). Mechanisms of support: Coping with loss in a major children's hospital. *Social Work in Health Care, 41*(1), 73-89.

Field, M. J., & Berman, R. E. (Eds.). (2003). *When children die: Improving end-of-life care for children and their families.* Washington, DC: Institute of Medicine of the National Academies.

Fitzgerald, M. (2005). The development of nociceptive circuits. *National Review of Neuroscience, 6*, 507-520.

Freyer, D. R. (2004). Care of the dying adolescent: Special considerations. *Pediatrics, 113*, 381-388.

Galloway, K. S., & Yaster, M. (2000). Pain and symptom control in terminally ill children. *Pediatric Clinics of North America, 47*, 711-746.

Geisel, T. S. (aka Dr. Seuss) (1954). *Horton hears a who!* New York: Random House.

Hain, R. D., Miser, A., Devins, M., & Wallace, W. H. (2005). Strong opioids in pediatric palliative medicine. *Pediatric Drugs, 7*, 1-9.

Hain, R., Weinsten, S., Oleske, J., Orloff, S. F., & Cohen, (2004). Holistic management of symptoms. In Carter, B. S. & Levetown, M. (Eds.) *Palliative care for infants, children, and adolescents: A practical handbook* (pp. 163-195). Baltimore: The Johns Hopkins University Press.

Himelstein, B. P., Hilden, J. M., Boldt, A.M., & Weissman, D. (2004). Pediatric palliative care. *New England Journal of Medicine, 350*(17), 1752-1762.

Krechel, S. W., & Bildner, J. (1995). CRIES: A new neonatal postoperative pain measurement score. Initial testing of validity and reliability. *Paediatric Anaesthesia, 5,* 53-61.

Lawrence, J., Alcock, D., McGrath, P., Kay, J., MacMurray, S. B., & Dulberg, C. (1993). The development of a tool to assess neonatal pain. *Journal of Neonatal Nursing, 12,* 59-66.

Leuthner, S. R. (2004). Palliative care of the infant with lethal anomalies. *Pediatric Clinics of North America, 51,* 747-759.

Massey, G. V., Pedigo, S., Dunn, N. L., Grossman, N. J., & Russell, E. C. (2002). Continuous lidocaine infusion for the relief of refractory malignant pain in a terminally ill pediatric cancer patient. *Journal of Pediatric Hematology and Oncology, 24,* 566-568.

McGrath, P. A., & Hillier, L. M. (2003). Modifying the psychologic factors that intensify children's pain and prolong disability. In N. L. Schechter, C. B. Berde, & M. Yaster (Eds.), *Pain in infants, children, and adolescents* (pp. 85-104). Philadelphia: Lippincott, Williams & Wilkins.

Merkel, S. I., Voepel-Lewis, T., Shayevitz, J. R., & Malviya, S. (1997). The FLACC: A behavioral scale for scoring postoperative pain in young children. *Pediatric Nursing, 23,* 293-297.

Nandi, R., & Fitzgerald, M. (2005). Opioid analgesia in the newborn. *European Journal of Pain, 9,* 105-108.

Perilongo, G., Rigon, L., Sainati, L., Cesaro, S., Carli, M., & Zanesco, L. (2001). Palliative and terminal care for dying children: Proposals for better care. *Medical and Pediatric Oncology, 37,* 59-61.

Pierucci, R. L., Kirby, R. S., & Leuthner, S. R. (2001). End-of-life care for neonates and infants: The experience and effects of a palliative care consultation service. *Pediatrics, 108,* 653-660.

Sahler, O. J., Frager, G., Levetown, M., Cohn, F. G., & Lipson, M. (2000). Medical education about end-of-life care in the pediatric setting. *Pediatrics, 104,* 575-584.

Saroyan, J. M., Schechter, W. S., Tresgallo, M. E., & Granowetter, L. (2005). Role of intraspinal analgesia in terminal pediatric malignancy. *Journal of Clinical Oncology, 23,* 1318-1321.

Serwint, J. R. (2004). One method of coping: Resident debriefing after the death of a patient. *Emergency Department, 145,* 229-234.

Subramaniam, K., Subramaniam, B., & Steinbrook, R. A. (2004). Ketamine as adjuvant analgesic to opioids: A quantitative and qualitative systematic review. *Anesthesia and Analgesia, 99,* 482-495.

Suresh, S., & Wheeler, M. (2002). Practical pediatric regional anesthesia. *Anesthesiology Clinics of North America, 20,* 83-113.

Suresh, S., & Anand, K. J. (2001). Opioid tolerance in neonates: A state-of-the-art review. *Paediatric Anaesthesia, 11,* 511-521.

Susman, E. (2005). Cancer pain management guidelines issued for children; adult guidelines updated. *Journal of the National Cancer Institute, 97,* 711-712.

Taddio, A., & Katz, J. (2004). Pain, opioid tolerance and sensitisation to nociception in the neonate. *Clinical Anaesthesiology, 18,* 291-302.

Thompson, K. L., & Varni, J. W. (1986). A developmental cognitive-biobehavioral approach to pediatric pain assessment. *Pain, 25,* 283-296.

Twycross, A. (1998). Children's cognitive level and perception of pain. *Professional Nurse, 14,* 35-37.

United Nations. (1989). Convention on the Rights of the Child, Article 12. High Commissioner of Human Rights. Retrieved September 11, 2005, from www.unhchr.ch/html/menu3/b/k2crc.htm.

Wolf, A. R. (1999). Pain, nociception and the developing infant. *Paediatric Anaesthesia, 9,* 7-17.

Wolfe, J., Grier, H. E., Klar, N., Levin, S. B., Ellenbogen, J. M., Salem-Schatz, S., et al. (2000). Symptoms and suffering at the end of life in children with cancer. *New England Journal of Medicine, 342,* 326-333.

■ CHAPTER 8 ■

Pharmacotherapy for Pain Control at the End of Life

By Arthur G. Lipman

In 1986, two important publications laid the foundation for the way clinicians now approach pain management in patients with advanced disease. One was the World Health Organization (WHO) booklet entitled *Cancer Pain Relief* (WHO, 1986). The other was the National Institutes of Health (NIH) Consensus Conference report entitled *The Integrated Approach to the Management of Pain*, which differentiated among acute pain, chronic pain associated with malignant disease (commonly termed chronic malignant pain), and pain not associated with malignant disease (chronic nonmalignant pain) (NIH, 1986). The broad, multimodal approaches advocated by both the WHO expert committee and the NIH Consensus Conference apply not just to cancer patients but also to the range of patients with advanced, irreversible disease seen in hospice care, including persons with AIDS, degenerative neurological diseases such as amyotrophic lateral sclerosis (ALS) and multiple sclerosis (MS), congestive heart failure, chronic obstructive pulmonary disease, end-stage organ system failure, and dementia. While interdisciplinary, multimodal care is optimal, pharmacotherapy is the cornerstone of most end-of-life symptom control. Hospice professionals must, therefore, be well versed in selecting and using appropriate drug therapy.

Pain intensity typically increases as life-limiting disease progresses with little or no adaptation. The increasing pain usually necessitates increases in the amount and types of analgesic therapy. It is not uncommon for people to think that increasing pain comes from the development of tolerance to opioid analgesics; however, increased analgesic requirements usually result from increasing or new pathology associated with the disorder that is causing the pain. Pain increases warrant titration of analgesics to provide adequate pain relief with tolerable side effects, but that is not always the best approach. In the 1990s, a common practice was to simply keep increasing opioid doses until the patient realized pain relief or the side effects became unacceptable. But opioids are not always the first-line or even the most effective drugs for all types of pain. More specific etiology-based therapy is a more effective strategy; this therapy may include pharmacological or nondrug treatments, as shown in Table 1.

Subsequent publications have further refined pain management strategies in end-of-life care. WHO published its most recent edition of *Cancer Pain Relief* in 1996. The American Pain Society publishes a very useful, pocket-sized clinical reference entitled *Principles of Analgesic Use in the Treatment of Acute Pain and Cancer Pain*; the fifth edition came out in 2003 (Ashburn & Lipman, 2003). The U.S. Department of Health and Human Services Agency for Healthcare Policy and Research (AHCPR) published an evidence-based clinical practice guideline on the management of cancer pain in 1994 (Jacox, Carr, Payne, Berde, Brietbart, et al., 1994). The AHCPR guideline contains excellent principles, but it has been superseded by the American Pain Society's *Guideline for the Management of Cancer Pain in Adults and Children* (Miaskowski, Cleary, Burney, Coyne, Finley, et al., 2005). The principles for managing cancer pain described in these documents apply to most hospice patients, for whom the focus is on comfort rather than rehabilitation or improving function.

Physical pain in end-of-life care is usually due to underlying physical pathology but also may result from treatment, such as surgery or radiotherapy. As they approach the end of life, many patients continue to experience pain from disorders that existed even before their life-threatening diagnoses (e.g., osteoarthritis and spinal compression fractures). Chronic

TABLE 1. FIRST-LINE THERAPY FOR END-OF-LIFE PAIN OF VARIOUS CAUSES

Etiology	First-Line Therapy
Bone	NSAID (plus opioid)
Neuropathic pain	Tricyclic antidepressant, antiepileptic drug, lidocaine
Infectious tissue damage	Anti-infective agents, incision and drainage
GI spasm	Anticholinergic agents
Constipation	Stimulating laxatives
Lymphedema	Physical therapy, massage

Note. Adapted from "Efficacy of Opioids in Cancer Pain Syndromes" (letter), by A. G. Lipman, 1995, *Pain, 63,* p. 135.

pain often is exacerbated by the inactivity and cognitive deterioration that are common in advanced disease and by the stressors and disturbed sleep these patients often experience. Emotional pain can markedly increase a patient's perception of pain; therefore, not just analgesics but also drugs to address emotional disorders and concurrent diseases may be needed to help control pain. Depression is common, but antidepressant pharmacotherapy takes several weeks to become fully effective and thus is usually not helpful in patients who enter hospice care with a life expectancy measurable in weeks rather than months. Central nervous system stimulants such as amphetamines and methylphenidate act promptly and can be helpful in managing depression at the end of life. Antianxiety drugs can be important adjuncts for some patients who experience serious anxiety as they approach the end of life. Stressors may include financial concerns and dysfunctional family or support group relationships; in these cases, counseling and family therapy often are more effective than drug therapy.

CHRONIC MALIGNANT PAIN MECHANISMS

Pharmacotherapy for pain in advanced disease should be based on the probable cause(s) of the pain whenever possible. The two major subtypes of pain are *nociceptive* and *neuropathic* pain, and the drug therapy for them differs.

Nociceptive insults can result from tumor pressure, inflammation, infection, ischemia, and other sequelae of progressive disease. This type of pain may be somatic or visceral. Somatic pain resulting from activation of primary afferent neurons in bone, skin, or soft tissue is usually described by the patient as sharp and localized. Visceral pain results from activation of visceral afferent neurons and is most commonly due to stretching or distention of organs or tissues within a body cavity. A common example in hospice care is liver capsule distention from hepatic cancer. Visceral pain is poorly localized and is usually described as dull and crampy. Visceral pain often is referred to different sites, making the source of the pain difficult to identify.

Nociceptive pain begins with peripheral physical insults activating (depolarizing) peripheral nociceptors, thereby initiating neurological messages that proceed to the spinal cord and thence to the brain, where they are perceived as pain (Hare, Voitanik, & Lipman, 2003). The nociceptive pathway from the periphery to the spinal cord is illustrated in Figure 1. Both peripherally acting agents—nonsteroidal anti-inflammatory drugs (NSAIDs), which act at the peripheral nociceptors, and centrally acting analgesics (e.g., opioids), which act in the dorsal horn of the spinal cord—are indicated and synergistic for nociceptive pain. These two analgesic drug classes are synergistic and mutually dose sparing.

Neuropathic pain is due to direct injury to peripheral or central nerves, which can result from tumor entrapment or compression or from ischemic, metabolic, chemical, or infectious mechanisms (Table 2). The nerve damage causes ectopic, spontaneous nerve discharges that produce pain that typically causes allodynia (exaggerated response to a non-noxious stimulus) and paresthesia or dysesthesia (tingling, pins and needles, a feeling of skin crawling).

NSAIDs are generally of little value in neuropathic pain management, because they act distally to the initiation site of the noxious stimuli on the

FIGURE 1. NOCICEPTIVE PATHWAY FROM THE PERIPHERY TO THE SPINAL CORD

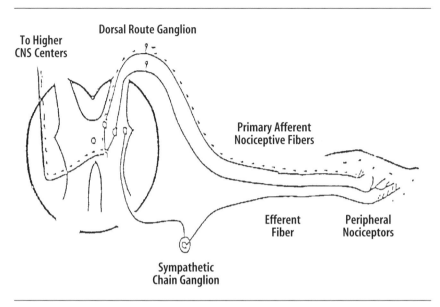

Source: Arthur G. Lipman

primary afferent sensory nerve fibers (Figure 1). Drugs that help to correct biochemical dysfunction in the affected nerves or that desensitize the neurons are the first-line therapy for neuropathic pain, as discussed below.

MULTIPLE PAINS

Patients with advanced disease frequently experience more than one type of pain concurrently; for example, acute pain, chronic pain not associated with their malignant disease, and breakthrough pain at various points in their disease process. Each must be addressed appropriately. Patients who are receiving end-of-life care commonly have more than one source of pain. A study of 100 consecutively admitted advanced cancer patients revealed that more than three quarters had pain of two or more different origins and over a third had four or more different pains (Twycross & Fairfield, 1982). Effective treatment of one pain may unmask another.

TABLE 2. CAUSES OF NEUROPATHIC PAIN SEEN IN END-OF-LIFE CARE

Disease-related

- Spinal cord compression
- Nerve entrapment

Treatment-related

- Phantom limb pain
- Chemotherapy
- Radiation therapy
- Surgery

Disease-related

- HIV neuropathy
- Cytomegalo virus
- Acute herpes zoster
- Post-herpetic neuralgia

Treatment-related

- Drug-induced neuropathy
- Radiation- or surgery-induced nerve damage

Note. From *Management of Chronic Pain in Patients with Cancer and HIV/AIDS* (CME Monograph 3), by the National Pain Education Council, 2002. Retrieved June 30, 2003, from www.npecweb.org/npec/CME.Guidelines/CME.monos.asp. Adapted with permission.

Many of these cancer patients' pains were not related to their cancers, and nearly half were of musculoskeletal origin. Such pain should be treated as any arthritic pain, not as severe cancer pain.

Breakthrough pain is common. This occurs when pain intensity increases unpredictably and is a part of the natural history of chronic pain. Breakthrough pain usually necessitates a supplemental dose of analgesic to cover the brief pain exacerbation, as shown in Figure 2. End-of-dose failure occurs when an analgesic is effective for a shorter than anticipated duration. This type of breakthrough pain often necessitates more frequent dosing. Sometimes increasing the dose suffices, because that extends the

Figure 2. Breakthrough Pain

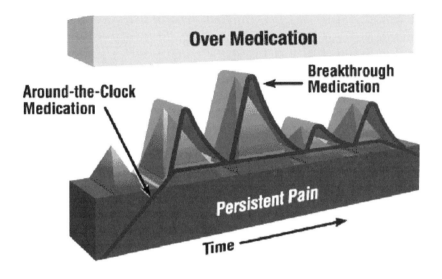

Note. From "Breakthrough Pain: Characteristics and Impact in Patients with Cancer Pain," by R. K. Portenoy, D. Payne, & P. Jacobson, 1999, *Pain*, p. 81. Copyright 1999 by *Pain*. Reprinted with permission.

time that the analgesic is at a therapeutic level. Patients with a large inflammatory component to their pain may report low pain intensity when they sit or lie still but increased pain when they move. This situation can be addressed by increasing anti-inflammatory pharmacotherapy.

Analgesics

The major classes of analgesics used in managing nociceptive pain are the prostaglandin inhibitors (acetaminophen and NSAIDs) and the opioids. The major drug classes used in neuropathic pain management are the tricyclic antidepressants (TCAs), antiepileptic drugs (AEDs), and local anesthetics, especially lidocaine. A paper published in the journal *Pain* concluded that opioids are not effective in neuropathic pain (Arner & Meyerson, 1989).

TABLE 3. EXAMPLES OF ADJUNCTIVE CO-ANALGESICS THAT MAY BE USEFUL IN END-OF-LIFE CARE

Drugs	Mechanisms of Action
Tricyclic antidepressants desipramine, amitriptyline	Inhibit monoamine reuptake
SSRI antidepressants sertraline, paroxetine	Improve affect (not analgesic)
Antiepileptic drugs gabapentin, pregabalin	Stabilize Na+ membranes
Trazodone	Facilitate sleep
Antihistamines	Facilitate sleep, treat allergies
Antianxiety agents	Decrease anxiety and stress
Central stimulants methylphenidate (Ritalin) dextroamphetamine modafenil (Provigil)	Decrease sedation

Source: Arthur G. Lipman

Subsequent work clearly demonstrated that opioids are often useful in neuropathic pain, although higher doses are sometimes needed than those used to manage nociceptive pain of similar intensity. Adjunctive drugs, sometimes called co-analgesics, also are needed to provide optimal pain management for many patients with end-of-life pain. These include antianxiety and antidepressant agents, sleeping aids, and central nervous system stimulants. Some drugs not generally considered to be analgesics but that may provide relief from pain are listed in Table 3.

PROSTAGLANDIN INHIBITORS

Prostaglandins are endogenous chemicals that are integrally involved in the transmission of noxious stimuli due to pain and inflammation. Prostaglandin formation in the human body requires the enzyme cyclooxygenase (COX). We now know that there are three isoforms of this enzyme—COX-1, COX-2, and COX-3. COX-3 was cloned in 2002 (Chandrasekharan et al., 2002). Aspirin and most other NSAIDs, such as ibuprofen, inhibit all three isoforms. Celecoxib (Celebrex) inhibits both COX-2 and COX-3 (i.e., it is COX-1 sparing). Acetaminophen inhibits only COX-3. That isoform exists only centrally (i.e., within the blood-brain barrier); therefore, it has no peripheral activity.

Inhibiting COX-1 disrupts several important homeostatic mechanisms (e.g., cytoprotection of the gastric mucosa) and does not produce analgesic or anti-inflammatory activity. Inhibition of COX-2 provides peripheral anti-inflammatory activity, and inhibition of COX-3 provides centrally mediated analgesia but no peripheral anti-inflammatory activity.

This explains why acetaminophen is an effective analgesic but lacks anti-inflammatory activity. Many end-of-life patients have painful inflammatory disorders for which NSAIDs are far more effective than acetaminophen. There is no reason to give both acetaminophen and an NSAID to a patient, because all NSAIDs inhibit COX-3, the mechanism through which acetaminophen acts. Most nonselective NSAIDs are markedly less expensive than the coxibs (COX-2 inhibitors), but the non-selective agents impair blood clotting by inhibiting platelet aggregation and thus present a risk of gastrointestinal ulceration. These adverse effects are minimally or not at all associated with coxibs. However, two of the three commercially available coxibs were withdrawn from the market recently as a result of the association of long-term use of these drugs with increased cardiovascular toxicity. The evidence now strongly suggests that any NSAID (including the over-the-counter NSAIDs ibuprofen, ketoprofen, and naproxen sodium) can increase cardiovascular risk, so toxicity is not unique to the coxibs. The mechanism is not fully clear, but any NSAID can increase blood pressure, which may, over time, be the major mechanism of cardiovascular toxicity. Clinicians should not allow cardiovascular concerns to keep them from using celecoxib rather than a nonselective NSAID when a coxib is indicated, but they must, of course, consider the issue in determining the risk:benefit ratio.

NEUROPATHIC PAIN DRUGS

Neuropathic pain is the major type of pain experienced by many degenerative neurological disease (MS, ALS) patients; it also occurs in over half of AIDS patients and at some point in the disease course of about 30% of cancer patients. Prostaglandin inhibitors have relatively little efficacy in neuropathic pain. The cause of this pain is direct damage to the primary afferent neuron, so agents that act on the damaged neuron constitute first-line pharmacotherapy.

Tricyclic antidepressants

Systematic reviews have consistently shown that TCAs are the drug of choice for this type of pain. TCAs inhibit reuptake of both serotonin and norepinephrine, increasing the levels of both of these chemicals in the nervous system. Both of these neurotransmitters are needed at sufficient levels for normal nerve transmission, and damaged nerves appear to require enhanced levels of both to function well. Most other types of antidepressants do not adequately elevate the levels of both neurotransmitters to be effective in neuropathic pain management. The commonly used selective serotonin reuptake inhibitor (SSRI) antidepressants do not raise norepinephrine levels, and venlafaxine (Effexor), the first serotonin-norepinephrine reuptake inhibitor (SNRI) antidepressant does not elevate both neurotransmitters adequately. The newer SNRI duloxetine (Cymbalta) does, but it is far more expensive than TCAs.

Because all TCAs are available generically, they are not aggressively marketed as the AEDs are, and many clinicians are unaware of the advantages of using them. They are very inexpensive, and they need to be dosed only once a day. The TCA doses used to manage neuropathic pain are only one third to one half the doses needed to treat depression, and the onset of effect is more rapid for pain relief than for depression: 1-3 weeks compared with 3-4 weeks. The dose-related side effects that have prevented clinicians from using TCAs to treat depression are a relatively small problem when the drugs are used for neuropathic pain, as long as the right TCA is selected.

The original TCAs have a tertiary side chain chemical structure that results in great anticholinergic and sedative side effects. The second-generation TCAs have a secondary side chain that lessens those effects.

TABLE 4. COMPARATIVE ANTICHOLINERGIC AND SEDATIVE EFFECTS OF TRICYCLIC ANTIDEPRESSANTS

Tricyclic Antidepressant Characteristics Tertiary Amines						
Drugs	Relative Anticholinergic Effects	Relative Sedative Effects	Relative Norepinephrine Reuptake Inhibition	Relative Serotonin Reuptake Inhibition	Relative Orthostatic Effects	Half-life in hours
amitriptyline	++++	++++	++	++++	++	30-45
imipramine	++	++	++	++++	+++	10-25
doxepin	++	+++	+	++++	++	8-25
clomipramine	+++	+++	++	++++	++	80-100
trimipramine	++	+++	+	+	++	7-30

Tricyclic Antidepressant Characteristics Secondary Amines						
Drugs	Relative Anticholinergic Effects	Relative Sedative Effects	Relative Norepinephrine Reuptake Inhibition	Relative Serotonin Reuptake Inhibition	Relative Orthostatic Effects	Half-life in hours
desipramine	+	+	++++	++	+	1-25
nortriptyline	++	++	++	+++	+	18-45
amoxapine	+++	++	+++	++	+	8-30
protriptyline	+++	+	++++	++	+	65-90

Note. Reprinted from "Analgesic Drugs for Neuropathic and Sympathetically Maintained Pain," by A. G. Lipman, 1996, *Clinics in Geriatric Medicine, p. 12*

Amitriptyline was the first TCA and is still the most commonly used drug in its class. However, it produces the most anticholinergic effects and sedation of all TCAs. The TCA of choice for neuropathic pain management is desipramine, because of its markedly lower side effect profile (illustrated in Table 4). Controlled trials have shown that desipramine is as effective as amitriptyline for neuropathic pain management. (Max, M.B., Lynch, S.A., Muir, J., Shoaf, S.E., Smoller, B., Dubner, R.) Effects of desipramine, amitriptyline, and fluoxetine on pain in diabetic neuropathy. (New England Journal of Medicine May, 1992.)

TCA dosing is normally started at 25 mg taken about an hour before bedtime to maximize the sedating effect of the drug. This dose is increased by 25 mg every three days until a maximum dose of 100 mg is reached. Most patients who respond to TCA therapy respond to doses in the 75-100 mg daily range. Higher doses may increase effectiveness but often produce unacceptable side effects. Frail elderly patients and those who are very sensitive to anticholinergic effects may be started at 10 mg about an hour before bedtime, with the dose increased by that amount about every 3 days until a maximum tolerated dose is reached or the dose reaches 100 mg. For neuropathic pain patients who have an extended life expectancy and a history of cardiac dysrhythmia, a baseline ECG may be indicated before initiating TCA therapy.

TCAs are not tolerated well by everyone, however. Side effects can be problematic, especially anticholinergic effects in patients with cardiac dysrythmias, men with benign prostatic hyperplasia, patients with severe constipation, and those with glaucoma. For patients with such problems, an AED may be the first-line drug for neuropathic pain. And because one third to one half of patients will not get adequate neuropathic pain relief from a TCA, the addition of (not replacement with) an AED is indicated after about 2 weeks of TCA therapy at the 100 mg daily dose.

ANTIEPILEPTIC DRUGS

Epileptic seizures are caused by spontaneous ectopic firing of motor neurons. Neuropathic pain is caused by spontaneous ectopic firing of damaged afferent sensory axons. Therefore, it is not surprising that the same types of drugs are sometimes useful for both conditions. All drugs that have antiepileptic efficacy have some effect on neuropathic pain, but the side effects of AEDs vary greatly. The best-studied AEDs for neuro-pathic pain are carbamazepine (Tegretol), specifically for trigeminal neuralgia, and gabapentin (Neurontin, generic), which is approved by the Food and Drug Administration (FDA) for post-herpetic neuralgia but has been used successfully for a broad range of neuropathic pain conditions. The new AED pregabalin (Lyrica) also has been well studied for neuro-pathic pain and appears to be as effective as gabapentin. Gabapentin must be administered three times a day to be effective, but pregabalin appears to be effective with twice-daily dosing. The cost is comparable, and both are

TABLE 5. NEWER ANTIEPILEPTIC DRUGS THAT HAVE BEEN USED TO TREAT NEUROPATHIC PAIN

Generic Name	Proprietary Name
Lamotrigine	Lamictal
Levetiracetam	Keppra
Oxcarbazepine	Trileptal
Pregabalin	Lyrica
Tiagabine	Gabitril
Topiramate	Topamax
Zonisamide	Zonegran

Source: Arthur G. Lipman

much more expensive than TCAs, which need to be administered only once daily. Neuropathic pain patients who do not respond to one AED may respond to another. The newer AEDs that have been used in neuropathic pain management are listed in Table 5. AEDs are nearly as effective as TCAs in the population of neuropathic pain patients, but some patients may respond better to one drug class than the other.

Another class of drugs that has similar efficacy to the TCAs and AEDs is the local anesthetics. Lidocaine is the local anesthetic most commonly used for neuropathic pain. It is effective intravenously, but continuous lidocaine infusions are extremely cumbersome and can produce toxicity. The oral local anesthetic analog cardiac drugs mexiletine (Mexitil) and tocainide (Tonocard) have been investigated as neuropathic pain agents. Mexiletine has been effective for some patients but has generally been disappointing. Tocainide is too toxic for this indication. Only with the introduction of the topical lidocaine patch (Lidoderm) has local anesthetic therapy for neuropathic pain gained popularity. Lidocaine patches are normally applied directly over the area of neuropathic pain and work for 12 hours on followed by a period of 12 hours off. Use of up to three full patches a day has been approved by the FDA for post-herpetic neuralgia, but such use is very expensive. An advantage of the lidocaine patch is that it can be cut with scissors before the backing is removed and it is applied, unlike transdermal fentanyl patches, which must never be cut. Therefore, for small areas of neuropathic pain, this medication can be cost-effective. The systemic levels of lidocaine achieved are very low, resulting in few side effects. Onset of activity may be seen within a week in some patients.

Because the mechanisms of action of these three drug classes differ, concurrent use of two or even all three may be synergistic.

Opioids are equally as effective as these drugs in many neuropathic pain patients and should certainly be considered if these three classes of medications provide inadequate analgesia.

OPIOIDS

Opioids are the most effective analgesics for most types of pain. The human body has several types of opioid receptors. The two types that are most often affected by pharmacotherapy are the mu (μ) and kappa (κ) receptors. Kappa agonists have a dose ceiling; that is, doses above a certain level provide no additional analgesia but do produce increasing side effects. Therefore, the kappa agonists are generally not useful in pain that increases over time, such as that most commonly seen in end-of-life care. Mu agonists, on the other hand, produce increasing analgesia as the dose is increased. There is not a priori upper dose limit for mu agonist opioids. The upper limit for any specific patient is the dose at which unacceptable side effect occur. Therefore, the mu agonists are the opioids of choice in hospice care. Approximate equianalgesic doses for available mu agonists are listed in Table 6.

Individuals may respond very differently to opioids. One reason for the variety of response is genetic polymorphism; that is, differences among people in the density of mu opioid subtypes causes different sensitivity to opioids (Jackson & Lipman, 2003). Thus, if a patient does not respond adequately to one opioid after multiple dose increases, it is wise to try another. Sometimes, patients who appear resistant to one opioid may respond dramatically to another; when changing opioids, use a conservative dose of the new drug initially (i.e., at least a 25% reduction from the equianalgesic dose).

TABLE 6. RELATIVE PROPERTIES OF COMMONLY USED OPIOID ANALGESICS

Drug	Approximate Equianalgesic Doses*	Dosing Interval	Duration of Action
Morphine**	30 mg (oral) 10 mg (parenteral)	Every 3-4 hours	3-4 hours
Codeine***	200 mg (oral), 120 mg to 130 mg (parenteral)	Every 3-4 hours	2-4 hours
Fentanyl	100 mcg (parenteral)	Every 1-2 hours (oral)	1-2 hours
Hydromorphone	7.5 mg (oral) 1.5 mg (parenteral)	Every 3-4 hours (PO)	2-4 hours
Hydrocodone	20 mg (oral)	Every 3-4 hours	4-5 hours
Levorphanol	4 mg (oral) 2 mg (parenteral)	Every 6-8 hours	4-5 hours
Meperidine[x]	300 mg (oral) 75 mg (parenteral)	Every 3 hours	2-4 hours
Methadone[xx]	10 mg (oral) 5 mg (parenteral)	Initial PO dosing TID-QID; initial parenteral dosing Q 6-8 hours. Dosing extends to every 8-12 hours after steady state is reached.	4-5 hours; 8-12 hours after reaching steady state; may take up to 10 days
Oxycodone	20 mg (oral)	Every 3-4 hours	2-4 hours
Oxymorphone	1 mg (parenteral)	Every 3-4 hours	4-6 hours

Note. PO = **[define]**; TID-QID = **[define?]**

*An equianalgesic dose is a dose of one analgesic that is equivalent in pain-relieving effects to another analgesic. This equivalence permits substitution of medications to avoid possible adverse effects of one of the drugs. The term is also applied to equivalent alternative dose sizes and routes of administration. Published tables vary in the suggested doses that are equianalgesic to morphine. Dosage must be titrated for each patient on the basis of clinical response. Because cross-tolerance among opioids is not complete, it is usually necessary to start with a lower than analgesic dose when changing drugs and retitrate to an analgesic level.

**With prn or single dose, the ratio of morphine is more commonly 6 to 1 rather than 3 to 1.

***Doses above 60 mg to 120 mg should not be used because of excessive nausea and constipation.

[x]Meperidine should be avoided in treating pain for more than 2 days because of its toxic metabolite, normeperidine, which can cause seizures or altered mental status.

[xx]Methadone should be used with extreme caution and only by experienced health care providers. Duration of analgesia can be shorter than the drug's half-life. Accumulation can occur, leading to life-threatening adverse side effects.

Opioids that should be avoided in managing pain in end-of-life care include meperidine; propoxyphene; the partial opioid agonist buprenorphine; and the mixed agonist/antagonists pentazocine, butorphanol, and nalbuphine (Jacox et al., 1994; Miaskowski et al., 2005). Meperidine should not be given because of its short half-life and the accumulation toxicity of normeperidine, which can result in seizures. Buprenorphine should be avoided because of its low efficacy and dose ceiling. Mixed agonist/antagonists also have a dose ceiling and may precipitate withdrawal in patients who are also taking pure opioid agonists because of competition for opioid receptors. Propoxyphene has low analgesic efficacy and can cause problematic side effects in patients with limited renal elimination capability. In fact, it is listed on the American Geriatrics Society's Beer's list as a drug that should not be given to elders (Sloane, Zimmerman, Brown, Ives, & Walsh, 2002). High doses of the pharmacologically long-acting opioids methadone and levorphanol should be used with caution because of their propensity to accumulate (Jackson & Lipman, 2003).

PRINCIPLES OF CHRONIC MALIGNANT PAIN MANAGEMENT

The World Health Organization expert committee defined five simple principles to be used in providing analgesia (WHO, 1986). These principles were validated through the evidence-based process that led to the AHCPR clinical practice guideline (Jacox et al., 1994). The principles and the evidence supporting them are described below.

Principle 1:
Provide Analgesia by the Oral Route Whenever Possible

When available and tolerated, the oral route should be used for analgesics. It is the most convenient route for most patients, is less of a burden than other routes on family caregivers, and is the most cost-effective method of drug administration. Furthermore, this simple route does not reinforce the "sick role" as do injections and other high-tech routes. Both immediate and controlled-release dosage forms are available to permit customized dosing regimens. However nausea and vomiting, decreased gastrointestinal function, and swallowing difficulty may limit the use of the oral route. When oral administration is not feasible, clinicians should consider other nonin-

TABLE 7. ALTERNATIVE NONINVASIVE ROUTES FOR OPIOID ADMINISTRATION

Route	Opioid	Comments
Sublingual (SL)	**Morphine** solution 1 ml SL held in the mouth for 10 minutes at pH 6.5 is 22% bioavailable. Lipophilicity increases absorption: **Methadone** is 34% bioavailable **Fentanyl** is 51% bioavailable	**Advantages** Avoid first-pass metabolism; lower cost than parenteral; comfort and ease for patient; effective in 15-25 minutes **Disadvantages** Low bioavailability; bitter taste; aftertaste; inconvenient for large doses; no fluids for ~15 minutes after dose
Buccal	**Fentanyl**	For breakthrough pain; same advantages and disadvantages as SL; transmucosal fentanyl lozenges are expensive
Inhalation	**Various**	**Advantages** Can be used in unconscious patients **Disadvantages** Cost (sterilization of drug, nebulizer rental); low bioavailability (12%-17%); no better than SL route in terminal dyspnea
Rectal	**Morphine** *Immediate-release oral tablets* peak 1 h; duration < 6 h *Controlled-release oral tablets* peak 5.4 h; duration 8-12 h *Oral solution* peak 0.5 h; duration 4-6 h *Rectal suppositories* peak 1.1 h; duration <6 h **Hydromorphone rectal suppositories** peak 1 h; duration 4-6 h **Methadone oral tablets** peak variable; duration 6-8 h **Oxycodone oral tablets and solution** peak 3.1 h; duration 8-12 h	**Advantages** Avoid first-pass metabolism; useful in temporary or terminal care; cost-benefit **Disadvantages** Patient's comfort may be compromised; absorption impaired by fecal material in colorectal area ■ inappropriate delivery vehicle ■ spontaneous expulsion that may occur with >10-15 ml of solution
Trans-dermal	**Fentanyl**	**Advantages** Encourages compliance; long acting (~ 72 hours) **Disadvantages** Expensive; difficult to titrate because of long time to steady-state serum levels; effects may continue for 12-24 hours after removing patch; levels may vary in rapidly progressing cachexia; effect may be increased by in tumor fever

Note. From "Chronic Malignant Pain," by K. L. Fakata, C. Miaskowsi, & A. G. Lipman, in A. G. Lipman (Ed.), *Pain Management for Primary Care Clinicians, 2004*, Bethesda, MD: saaaAmericanSociety of Health-System Pharmacists vasive routes before injections (Table 7). These include rectal, transmucosal, and transdermal administration. The rectal route can be useful for temporary or terminal care if the rectal mucosa is relatively intact and this route is esthetically acceptable to the patient and family caregivers. This route is not usually good for long-term administration because of rectal irritation from repeated dosing. Although the rectal and lower colonic mucosa have limited surface area for drug absorption, absorption is adequate when the dosage form is placed just above the rectal sphincter; this placement allows absorption from the lower and middle rectal veins that bypass the portal circulation. Inserting the dosage form higher into the rectal vault favors absorption by the superior rectal vein that empties into the portal vein, allowing first-pass metabolism that markedly decreases the effect of the dose.

Sublingual, buccal, and cheek pouch (lingual) administration of small volumes (not >1 ml under the tongue or a few ml in the cheek or lip pouch) permit a drug solution or sublingual tablets (not regular, compressed tablets) to be absorbed through the oral mucosa. More lipophilic drugs are better absorbed from this route. The sublingual route is most efficient, but part of the dose normally trickles down the throat and is absorbed through normal enteral mechanisms if it is not inactivated by gastric fluid; therefore, it is difficult to estimate the equivalence between swallowed and sublingual doses. Normally, start with approximately the same dose and titrate according to response.

Oral transmucosal fentanyl citrate lozenges (Actiq) are an FDA-approved transmucosal dosage form for the management of breakthrough cancer pain in patients who are tolerant to opioid therapy for their persistent cancer pain. About 25% of the fentanyl dose is rapidly absorbed transmucosally, and about 75% of the dose is swallowed. About a quarter of the swallowed dose is slowly absorbed from the intestines, producing net bioavailability of about 50%. This dosage form can be very useful for patients whose breakthrough pain escalates rapidly, but it is expensive. Most patients do well with inexpensive oral immediate-release tablets for breakthrough pain. While tablets take 30 to 45 minutes to work, patients commonly report relief within a few minutes, probably because experience has taught them that they will get relief after a dose of analgesic. When patients relax, knowing that they have received a dose of analgesic, the relaxation reduces pain perception.

Transdermal administration is convenient, and the commercially available, long-acting fentanyl patch favors adherence (compliance). While most patients get 72 hours of relief from a patch, experience shows that one fifth to one quarter experience end-of-dose failure before that time, necessitating the application of a fresh patch every 48 hours. Extemporaneously compounded transdermal opioid and NSAID formulations lack adequate efficacy and safety data and are not recommended.

Principle 2: Individualize Dosing

Different patients may respond very differently to the same opioid, even when the etiology of their pain and its intensity are similar. A common axiom in opioid dosing is "the dose that works is the dose that works." Interpatient variability in response to opioids should be expected. Published dosage tables are based on population averages and may not apply to an individual patient. Titration to response is the only reliable method to determine the best dose for each patient.

In a study of 955 advanced cancer patients admitted to an inpatient hospice program, investigators were able to titrate all of the patients to comfort using a simple aqueous morphine solution administered every 4 hours. The doses ranged from 2.5 mg to 180 mg per day (Twycross & Fairfield, 1982).

Principle 3: By the Ladder

The 1986 WHO publication describes a three-step analgesic ladder (Figure 3). The first step of the ladder is acetaminophen (if inflammation does not contribute to the pain) or an NSAID; the second step is a low dose of an opioid plus NSAID; and the third step is a higher dose of opioid plus NSAID. On all steps, adjuvants (e.g., antidepressants, anxiolytics) should be administered as needed.

A "fourth step" for pain relief might include pain management techniques such as cognitive behavioral therapy, nerve blocks, implantable devices, palliative chemotherapy, and palliative irradiation.

FIGURE 3. WORLD HEALTH ORGANIZATION ANALGESIC LADDER

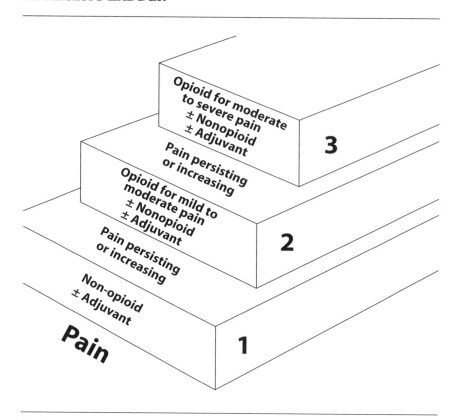

Note. From *Cancer Pain Relief* (No. 804), 1986, Geneva: World Health Organization.
Copyright WHO. Reprinted with permission.

STEP 1

Nonopioid analgesic plus adjuvant for the treatment of mild pain that is persisting or increasing.

Mild pain is that which elicits a patient pain intensity rating of 1-3 on a 1-10 pain intensity scale in which zero represents no pain and 10 the worst pain the patient can imagine. Pharmacotherapy in Step 1 includes acetaminophen and NSAIDs. For around-the-clock pain relief, acetaminophen should be dosed at 1 g four times daily. Lower doses are necessary in the presence of frank liver disease, but there is no evidence that lower doses should be used in elderly patients with reasonable hepatic function. NSAIDs are beneficial in nociceptive pain when there is inflammation. The COX-2 selective NSAID celecoxib can be used far more safely than the nonselective NSAIDs in patients with history of GI ulcers or those who have bleeding problems. Tramadol is another option for patients in Step 1 of the WHO ladder who cannot tolerate NSAIDs. Tramadol is a weak mu agonist (mild opioid activity) that also inhibits the reuptake of norepinephrine and serotonin. Tramadol can cause nausea and should be titrated slowly as tolerated to a maximum of 400 mg in 24 hours.

Step 2

Opioid for mild to moderate pain added to a nonopioid analgesic with or without adjunctive therapy.

Moderate pain is the intensity consistent with a patient pain intensity rating of 4-7 on a pain intensity scale of 1-10. This therapy typically consists of relatively low-dose, short-acting agents in combination with (not in place of) acetaminophen or NSAIDs. Start opioid-naive patients with moderate to severe pain at this step. Combination opioid formulations have a dose ceiling because of the nonopioid component. If these agents are no longer sufficient to treat moderate to severe pain in the opioid-naive patient, proceed to Step 3.

Step 3

Opioid for moderate to severe pain with or without nonopioid analgesic or adjuvant medications.

Severe pain is that resulting in a patient pain intensity rating of 7-10 on a pain intensity scale of 1-10. The opioids used in this step are pure mu agonists, and high doses are often required as disease progresses. If the dose causes excessive side effects, a decrease of 20% may be warranted. At Step 3, consistent dosing is required and a modified-release or pharmacologically long-acting opioid for around-the-clock pain control is usually preferred. The patient should also have an immediate-release opioid to use as a rescue dose for breakthrough pain. An appropriate rescue dose might be one half of the every-4-hour dose (one sixth of an every-12-hour dose) every 2 hours for breakthrough pain. If more than two or three rescue doses per day are required for more than two or three days, increase the regularly scheduled dose by half or titrate the long-acting opioid by adding the total of the rescue doses used in a 24-hour period.

Some guidelines no longer advocate the three-step analgesic ladder, because some insurance companies consider this a stepped approach to therapy and incorrectly assume that all patients should be started on the first step. Patients should be started on the step needed for effective pain control with minimal side effects. For many advanced disease patients, Step 3 may be the appropriate level at which to start therapy.

PRINCIPLE 4: ADMINISTER ANALGESICS ON A REGULAR SCHEDULE (BY THE CLOCK)

When the noxious stimulus causing the pain is ongoing, administration of analgesics on an around-the-clock schedule provides consistent and adequate pain control. Oral controlled-release opioid dosage forms provide continuous delivery over 8-24 hours. Anxiety, depression, and sleep disturbance are associated with inadequate pain control; consistent dosing often lessens these confounding disorders. In addition, patients should be able to receive short-acting dosage forms for breakthrough pain.

PRINCIPLE 5: USE ADJUVANTS

Pain associated with end-of-life care is not a single symptom; it is part of a symptom complex, as illustrated in Figure 4. Appropriate adjuvant medications can improve patients' quality of sleep, lessen depression and anxiety, and manage opioid-induced side effects such as nausea and sedation. Adjuvant analgesics including tricyclic antidepressants, anticonvulsants, and lidocaine are indicated for neuropathic pain as described below.

Expect constipation with regularly scheduled opioid analgesia. This effect is due to activation of opioid receptors in the colon, which inhibits peristalsis; therefore, stool softeners alone are usually inadequate. Chemically induced peristalsis is needed. Stimulating laxatives such as senna are the laxatives of choice. For patients who do not respond to such stimulants, methylnaltrexone and alvimopan are peripherally acting opioid antagonists that should be considered (Camilleri, 2005; Yuan, 2004). At the time of this writing, these drugs were still investigational, with approval anticipated within a year or two. Peripherally acting opioid

FIGURE 4. CHRONIC PAIN SYMPTOM COMPLEX

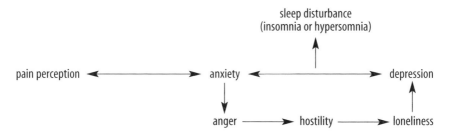

Chronic Pain Symptom Complex

Note. From "Drug Therapy in the Management of Pain," by A. G. Lipman, 1990, *British Journal of Pharmaceutical Practice, 12,*. Copyright *British Journal of Pharmaceutical Practice*. Reprinted with permission.

antagonists do not cross the blood-brain barrier and, therefore, will not reverse opioid analgesia.

EFFECTIVENESS OF THE WHO THREE-STEP LADDER

Medical records from 2,118 patients who received care for over 140,478 days were examined to define the effectiveness of this approach to cancer pain management. The analgesics in Step 1 of the ladder were effective for only 11% of treatment days; Step 2 analgesia was needed for 31% of the days; and Step 3 analgesia was needed for 49% of the days (Zech, Grond, Lynch, Hertel, & Lehmann, 1995). Palliative anticancer drugs were included in the analgesic regimen of 42% of the patients, nerve blocks in 8%, physical therapy in 5%, and psychotherapy in 3%. Over three-quarters (76%) of the patients rated their pain relief as good, and an additional 12% rated their comfort as satisfactory. In their final days of life, 84% of the patients rated their pain as moderate or less.

Thus, this simple approach to pain management in advanced disease provided satisfactory or better pain relief in nearly 90% of the patients studied.

BARRIERS TO EFFECTIVE ANALGESIC THERAPY

Patients and family members, health care professionals, and the health care system can all be barriers to effective pain management. Many patients, families, and professionals fear that opioid analgesics will cause unacceptable side effects or will impair patients' ability to communicate. Many fear addiction, physical dependence, and tolerance. None of these concerns should be barriers to the appropriate use of opioids.

Some patients deny or inaccurately report pain because they fear becoming a burden. Many fear that tolerance will develop if they use opioids too soon, causing intractable pain later in the course of their disease. Patients may inconsistently report pain to different health care professionals; for example, high pain complaints to a nurse and relative denial of pain to the physician. This can delay adequate pain therapy. On the other hand, some professionals are uncomfortable using opioids to relieve pain—they may fear detriment to the patient or scrutiny by regulatory agencies.

Pain management education is minimal in many health profession training programs. Clinicians who feel that their training is inadequate to enable them to treat their patients' pain should consider referral to others who are more experienced in this type of practice.

Another obstacle is reimbursement from managed care organizations. Insurance programs may only pay for a set amount of pain medications they consider to equal a one-month supply, not taking into account that chronic pain management dose requirements are not static. Depending on the opioid dose and the route of administration, the out-of-pocket expense to the patient can be large. Some managed care programs also resist covering psychosocial treatment that is an important aspect of CMP management.

CONCLUSION

Severe pain occurs at some stage in many progressive diseases, not just cancer and AIDS. Chronic pain may be exacerbated by acute pain episodes, and it may include both nociceptive and neuropathic components. Pain can be expected to worsen as the disease progresses, and aggressive treatment with both pharmacologic and nonpharmacologic approaches is warranted to minimize suffering. The WHO ladder provides a simple but effective guide to analgesic pharmacotherapy; however, it is important to individualize treatment to meet each patient's pain requirements. Clinicians should remain aware of potential barriers to adequate pain relief and should assess and reassess pain with valid assessment tools. Pain is not only physical but includes emotional, social, spiritual, financial, and existential components. With attention to detail and consultation and referral when needed, most pain encountered in end-of-life care can be managed to the degree necessary for patients to live their remaining days with dignity while being able to communicate effectively, say their good-byes, and do the other work necessary at the end of life. ■

Arthur G. Lipman is Professor of Pharmacotherapy, Adjunct Professor of Anesthesiology, Director of Clinical Pharmacology, Pain Management Center, at the University of Utah. Formerly, Dr. Lipman served on the faculty at Yale University Medical and Graduate Nursing Schools.

Dr. Lipman served on both the Acute Pain Management and Cancer Pain Management Guidelines Panels of the U.S. Public Health Service Agency for Health Care Policy and Research. He was an investigator on the original NIH-sponsored demonstration of hospice care and has been a hospice consultant, board member and president during the past 30 years. His professional service includes co-chair of the American Pain Society Arthritis Pain Management Clinical Guidelines Panel, American Cancer Society National Advisory Group on Cancer Pain Relief, American Pain Society Analgesic Regulatory Affairs Committee and the Ethics Task Force of the American Pain Society and American Academy of Pain Medicine. He co-chaired the American Pain Society Analgesic Principles 2003 revision committee.

Dr. Lipman is founding editor of the Journal of Pain & Palliative Care Pharmacotherapy *(indexed in Medline/PubMed). He also has been editor of the Research Update and Palliative Care departments of the* American Pain Society Bulletin. *Dr. Lipman has published five books and over 150 articles, chapters, and monographs plus over 300 reviews.*

REFERENCES

Arner, S., & Meyerson, B. A. (1989). Lack of analgesic effect of opioids on neuropathic and idiopathic forms of pain. *Pain, 39*, 243-246.

Ashburn, M. A., & Lipman, A. G. (Eds.). (2003). *Principles of analgesic use in the treatment of Acute Pain and Cancer Pain* (5th ed.). Glenview, IL: American Pain Society.

Bernabei, R., Gambassi, G., Lapane, K., et al. (June 1998). Management of pain in elderly patients with cancer. SAGE Study Group, systematic assessment of geriatric drug use via epidemiology. *Journal of the American Medical Association, 279*(23), 1877-1882.

Camilleri, M. (2005). Alvimopan, a selective peripherally acting mu-opioid antagonist. *Neurogastroenterology and Motility, 17*, 157-165.

Chandrasekharan, N. V., Dai, H., Roos, K. L., Evanson, N. K., Tomsik, J., Elton, T. S., et al. (October 2002). COX-3, a cyclooxygenase-1 variant inhibited by acetaminophen and other analgesic/antipyretic drugs: Cloning, structure, and expression. *Proceedings of the National Academy of Sciences, USA, 99*(21), 13926-13931. Epub 2002 Sep 19. http://www.pnas.org/ accessed September 15, 2005

Fakata, K. L., Miaskowsi, C., & Lipman, A. G. (2004). Chronic malignant pain. In A. G. Lipman (Ed.), *Pain management for primary care clinicians.* Bethesda, MD: American Society of Health-System Pharmacists

Hare, B. D., Voitanik, S., & Lipman, A. G. (2003). Pathophysiology of pain. In A. G. Lipman (Ed.), *Pain management for primary care clinicians.* Bethesda, MD: American Society of Health-System Pharmacists

Jackson, K. C., & Lipman, A. G. (2003). Opioid analgesics. In A. G. Lipman (Ed.), *Pain management for primary care clinicians.* Bethesda, MD: American Society of Health-System Pharmacists

Jacox, A., Carr, D. B., Payne, R., Berde. C. B., Brietbart, S., Cain, J. M. et al. (1994). *Management of cancer pain: Clinical practice guideline* (AHCPR Publication Number 94-0592). Rockville, MD: Agency for Healthcare Policy and Research.

Lipman, A. G. (1990). Drug therapy in the management of pain. *British Journal of Pharmaceutical Practice, 12,* 22-29.

Lipman, A. G. (1995). Efficacy of opioids in cancer pain syndromes (letter). *Pain, 63,* 135.

Lipman, A. G. (1996). Analgesic drugs for neuropathic and sympathetically maintained pain. *Clinics in Geriatric Medicine, 12,* 501-515.

Miaskowski, C., Cleary, J., Burney, R. Coyne, P. J., Finley R., Foster, R., et al. (2005). *Guideline for the management of cancer pain in adults and children.* Glenview, IL: American Pain Society.

National Institutes of Health. (1986). *The integrated approach to the management of pain.* NIH Consensus Development Conference. *Journal of Pain and Symptom Management, 2*(1), 35-44.

National Pain Education Council. (2002). *Management of chronic pain in patients with cancer and HIV/AIDS* (CME Monograph 3). Retrieved June 30, 2003, from www.npecweb.org/npec/CME.Guidelines/CME.monos.asp.

Portenoy, R. K., Payne, D., & Jacobsen, P. (1999). Breakthrough pain: Characteristics and impact in patients with cancer pain. *Pain, 81*(1-2), 129-134.

Sloane, P. D., Zimmerman, S., Brown, L. C., Ives, T. J., & Walsh, J. F. (2002). Inappropriate medication prescribing in residential care/assisted living facilities. *Journal of the American Geriatrics Society, 50,* 1001-1011.

Twycross, R. G., & Fairfield, S. (November 1982). Pain in far-advanced cancer. *Pain, 14*(3), 303-310.

World Health Organization. (1986). *Cancer pain relief.* Geneva: Author.

World Health Organization. (1996). *Cancer pain relief with a guide to opioid availability* (2nd ed.). Geneva: Author.

World Health Organization. (1990). *Cancer pain relief and palliative care* (No. 804). Geneva: Author.

Yuan, C. S. (2004). Clinical status of methylnaltrexone, a new agent to prevent and manage opioid-induced side-effects. *The Journal of Supportive Oncology, 2,* 111-117.

Zech, D. F., Grond, S., Lynch, J., Hertel, D., & Lehmann, K.A. (October 1995). Validation of World Health Organization guidelines for cancer pain relief: A 10-year prospective study. *Pain, 63*(1), 65-76.

CHAPTER 9

Approaches to End-of-Life Pain Management

By Janet L. Abrahm

What is quality care for patients at the end of life? According to surveys of patients and their families, quality includes comfort, a sense of control and dignity, relieving burdens on loved ones, strengthening and completing relationships with significant others, and avoiding prolongation of the dying process (Singer, Martin, & Kelner, 1999). It is not enough to provide complete relief of troublesome symptoms if, in so doing, we create sedated patients who cannot accomplish these tasks. Expert relief of pain requires practitioners to use a range of modalities to achieve a level of relief that the patient finds satisfactory but that also enables patients to be cognitively intact and recognizably themselves. Physical pain, after all, is only one of the dimensions of suffering that patients report to us as "pain." Psychological distress, social and financial concerns, and spiritual and existential crises all cause suffering, and all must be addressed if we are to alleviate the pain of our dying patients and ameliorate the suffering of their loved ones (Ferrell & Rhiner, 1991).

Hospice programs contain the ideal mix of personnel to address all aspects of suffering. They include interdisciplinary teams of physicians, nurses, social workers, chaplains, and specially trained volunteers, all of whom assess and try to alleviate suffering and pain in all its forms. This volume similarly addresses each of the dimensions of pain and the various barriers to its relief (psychological, spiritual, social, cultural, and political). Other authors review the physiology of pain, pain assessment at the end of life, the challenges of assessment in demented patients, pharmaceutical strategies, complementary therapies, and the role of psychological and spiritual distress in the experience of pain. In this chapter, I will review crucial pitfalls in pain assessment and management in patients at the end of life and novel techniques that can help us overcome some of the most intractable pain problems.

PITFALLS IN PAIN ASSESSMENT AND MANAGEMENT

You have to see the pain to treat the pain. As simple as this seems, it presents one of the major barriers to relief of pain at the end of life. Both clinicians and families who are unfamiliar with the "look" of chronic pain fail to recognize it when it occurs. Most people, when asked to think of what a patient in pain "looks like," conjure up the image of a person who has acute pain from an injury, or a headache, or a heart attack. The person is grimacing, moaning, perhaps crying and, when examined carefully, has an elevated pulse and blood pressure. These findings occur when the autonomic nervous system is activated, as happens when someone develops acute pain. But, over time, the nervous system accommodates to the painful stimulus, and these findings disappear. Without them, it may be hard for a clinician or a family member to believe the patient's pain complaint.

But imagine, instead, a patient we'll call Mrs. Sanders, a 34-year-old woman with recurrent refractory ovarian carcinoma with a mass that is invading the bones of her sacrum and pelvis. She characterizes her pain as aching and gnawing in her pelvis and burning in her buttocks and perineum. She is unable to sit comfortably and is even uncomfortable lying in bed. This description reveals that Mrs. Sanders' pain is both somatic (from her bones) and neuropathic, from the cancer invading the nerves in her sacral plexus. This pain has been there for a long time, so while she may report a pain level of 9/10, she is unlikely to be grimacing or crying and will have normal blood pressure and pulse. There are other diagnostic signs that help us quantitfy her distress. She moves little (protecting her painful buttocks and pelvis), sleeps badly, has a short temper, and is uncharacteristically withdrawn and depressed. Clinicians and families must recognize these more subtle signs if they are to help ameliorate patients' chronic pain.

Mrs. Sanders' disease has created much more than physical discomfort for her. It has changed her family, social, and spiritual life. She can't join her family for meals or go to church. She has had to give up playing with her children (5 and 9 years old) and attending her monthly book club. Her parents have moved into her home to help her while her husband is at work. She has, in effect, lost her roles in the community and her role as caregiver for her family. Relieving her pain may help her regain some of these roles and make her more whole. In so doing, her clinicians may relieve her suffering even as her cancer progresses (Cassell, 2004).

NONPHARMACOLOGIC THERAPIES

Too heavy a reliance on the very effective drugs we now have to treat pain can cause us to lose sight of other useful techniques that can help patients like Mrs. Sanders. Even if she were in an acute care setting or rehabilitation hospital, her family could lessen her distress by personalizing her room—playing her favorite music; adding pictures of family, trips, or pets; or bringing bedding from home. When at home or in the hospital, Mrs. Sanders also might get relief from manipulative and body-based methods of pain control, such as hot or cold wraps or gels, massage therapy, and careful positioning (Abrahm, 2005).

Spiritual and psychological counseling would also be of great benefit to her. In addition, by working with a cognitive-behavioral therapist, she could learn mindfulness meditation, relaxation therapy, or hypnosis to help her deal with her pain.

Mindfulness is one of the three general types of meditation, along with concentrative and contemplative. In concentrative meditation, the practitioner focuses on a word, mantra, or image. Prayer is a typical type of contemplative meditation. Vipassana and Soto Zen are forms of mindfulness meditation, as is the method of Jon Kabat-Zinn, who uses mindfulness in his clinical practice with patients who have pain, stress, or cardiovascular disease (Kabat-Zinn, 1990).

Relaxation therapy can be used alone or as an induction in hypnosis, a powerful cognitive technique for patients with pain. Through use of hypnosis, patients can be taught to regain control over situations from which much control has been lost. Hypnosis itself is not therapy, but therapy takes place while the patient is in trance. Almost everyone can experience a clinically useful trance to diminish insomnia, anxiety, feelings of helplessness, loss of control, nausea, or pain. Patients use metaphor and imagery while in trance to modify their experience of the distressing syndrome. Patients like Mrs. Sanders, who have chronic "meaningless" pain, can learn how to "put the pain away, in a trunk in the attic" and experience only today's pain, not amplified by the memory of yesterday's or the fear of tomorrow's. The "volume" of the pain can be turned down; the hurtful "color" of it changed to a more comforting one. Practitioners of hypnosis can make tapes to help patients enter into and stay in trance to do the work they'd like to do there. Patients also can dissociate the painful part so that it is "not theirs" or distract themselves in trance by "going to" a favorite vacation spot. Other distraction techniques vary from something as simple as using earphones or headphones to play music or a book on tape during a procedure to head-mounted virtual reality devices (Abrahm, 2005).

Alternative medical systems offer many benefits for patients with advanced disease. They embrace theories that differ from those of standard medical practice regarding what promotes health of the mind, body, and spirit; what causes illness; and how health and balance can be regained. Acupuncture is a part of classic Chinese medicine that has documented efficacy for pain, dyspnea, and nausea (Weiger, Smith, Boon, Richardson, Kaptchuk, et al., 2002). Yoga is "a discipline that nurtures the union of body, mind, and spirit and emphasizes that as human beings we are part of a larger whole and not just isolated individuals. One of the underlying beliefs of yoga is that there is more right with us than wrong with us and that, despite experiences of illness or disease, we are more than our illness or disease" (Ott, 2002, p.81). Of the eight major branches of yoga, hatha yoga is the most often used in the medical context. Patients like Mrs. Sanders who are bedridden can use specially modified asanas (physical postures). The effects on anxiety, strength, flexibility, and breathing would be particularly useful for her. Complementary therapies are reviewed in chapter 10.

Music and art therapists can work with Mrs. Sanders and her family to minimize her suffering and teach her how to express in ways other than words the emotions she is feeling and what she would like her loved ones to remember about her.

PITFALLS IN NEUROPATHIC PAIN MANAGEMENT

But the kind of pain that Mrs. Sanders has is very unlikely to respond to nonpharmacologic or complementary therapies alone. She has severe neuropathic pain, one of the most difficult pain syndromes to treat. She will need opioids and neuropathic adjuvant agents. It is very easy to cause serious side effects with these drugs, and it is very important to be skillful in using a variety of available agents when side effects do occur. The following scenario illustrates the pitfalls that occurred in Mrs. Sanders' care.

Mrs. Sanders recently enrolled in her local hospice program. Her nurse, Joyce, found her to be in 9/10 pain. Mrs. Sanders told her hospice social worker, Bruce, that she has begun feeling like a burden to everyone, hopeless and helpless. Bruce is concerned that she has developed depression, one of the most common sequelae of uncontrolled pain (Block, 2000). Mrs. Sanders told the hospice chaplain, Katherine, that lately she asks herself what she could have done that was so terrible that God is punishing her with this intractable pain. To lessen her physical, mental, and spiritual anguish, Mrs. Sanders needs better control of her pain.

Joyce has been working with the oncology team to find a better pain regimen for Mrs. Sanders. Her husband reports that she has been moaning more lately, and it is hard for her to engage in conversation. She is currently taking ibuprofen 600 mg three times a day for the pain from her bony metastases, along with omeprazole to protect her stomach, and laxatives. She is also taking a sustained-release morphine preparation, which has been increased to 300 mg every eight hours. Her husband gives her 90 mg of a concentrated morphine elixir (50 mg per ml) as often as every three hours when he thinks she is in pain. He gave her six doses yesterday. She is sleeping badly, having nightmares.

Joyce and the oncology team decide to increase Mrs. Sanders' sustained-release morphine by about 50%, to 500 mg every eight hours (900 mg + 450 mg = 1350 mg), with a 150 mg rescue dose (i.e., 10% of the total daily dose) (Miaskowski, Cleary, Burney, Coyner, Finley, et al., 2005), and they added gabapentin 100 mg by mouth daily as an initial dose to minimize the sedation that the drug often induces. They planned to raise her dose to 300 mg three times a day over the next two weeks. Joyce was gratified that Mrs. Sanders' pain levels decreased to about 5/10 on this regimen, which was satisfactory to her.

However, a week later, Mrs. Sanders' husband called to report that his wife was sleeping even less, seemed very restless, and was much more confused. Over the weekend, he had been giving her the immediate-release morphine every three hours for increased back pain, but this morning she had begun to moan and he didn't know what to do. Everywhere he touched her seemed to be painful, and she was seeing people in the room whom others didn't see. Even if this meant she was dying, he wanted help in relieving her distress. Joyce immediately offered to admit Mrs. Sanders to the hospital for evaluation on her inpatient hospice benefit.

What was happening to Mrs. Sanders? How can her pain be controlled? Mrs. Sanders was using a good adjuvant for her bone pain (ibuprofen), but she and her husband tried to treat her uncontrolled neuropathic pain with increasing doses of morphine. Adjuvants such as gabapentin are usually needed to treat this pain (Lussier, Huskey, & Portenoy, 2004), and it would be days to weeks before she achieved therapeutic levels of gabapentin. To relieve neuropathic pain until adequate levels of gabapentin are reached, we use corticosteroids. We usually start with a 10 mg dexamethasone oral dose, followed by 4 to 6 mg four times a day for a day or two. If there is a dramatic response, which often occurs, we then rapidly taper the dexamethasone to the lowest tolerable dose while we gradually raise the gabapentin doses to a minimum of 300 mg three times a day. For some patients, adding another neuropathic pain adjuvant, a tricyclic antidepressant such as nortriptyline or amitriptyline at bedtime, enhances sleep and provides additional pain relief (Abrahm, 2005; Lussier et al., 2004). For patients whose neuropathic pain is not from chemotherapy or cancer but is due to an alcoholic or diabetic peripheral neuropathy, tramadol alone can provide excellent relief.

When she was admitted, Mrs. Sanders moaned continuously. In addition, she cried aloud whenever she was touched (even on her arms, where she had no metastases) and when she was rolled over to change her bedding. She had severe myoclonus and visual hallucinations, and was fearful of family or nurses offering her medications, because she thought they were trying to poison her. She was reluctant to interact with her caregivers; on careful questioning, it was clear that she was distracted, disoriented, and had disorganized thinking. She was slightly dehydrated but had normal calcium, glucose, and electrolytes, and was not infected or hypoxic.

Opioid-Induced Neurotoxicity

Mrs. Sanders had all the hallmarks of opioid-induced neurotoxicity. Opioid-induced neurotoxicity can include myoclonus (which can progress to seizures, especially with renal insufficiency), hyperalgesia, and delirium. The moaning was actually a manifestation of a developing delirium, but her husband had incorrectly interpreted it as uncontrolled pain, which he treated with repeated doses of morphine (Coyle, Breitbart, Weaver, & Portenoy, 1994).

The myoclonus, the allodynia (pain on her arms from a nonpainful stimulus), and the hyperalgesia (severe pain when being rolled, which was usually only a mildly painful stimulus) were probably due to elevated levels of morphine and its metabolites: morphine-3 and morphine 6-glucuronide (M-3-G and M-6-G). Her delirium was manifested by the acute onset of visual hallucinations, paranoia, distraction, disorientation, and disorganized thinking (Breitbart et al., 1997). Other manifestations of delirium include reduced level of consciousness, disturbance of the sleep/wake cycle, and decreased or increased psychomotor activity (Breitbart et al., 1997).

Mrs. Sanders' admitting team recognized that she had a delirium induced by the morphine. Delirium, if caused by opioids and dehydration, reverses in about 50% of patients (Lawlor et al., 2000). The team chose to hydrate her to clear the toxic morphine metabolites and to change her opioids. Changing opioids to diminish neurotoxicity is called "opioid rotation" (Indelicato & Portenoy, 2002). Studies of its efficacy are observational and uncontrolled (Quigley, 2005), but the studies and anecdotal evidence support the practice.

The team added lorazepam 1 mg intravenously every six hours as needed for her myoclonus, planning to add the neurontin back when she was able to take oral medications. A hydromorphone drip was begun at 1 mg/hour. Nothing specific was added for her delirium, because she was less agitated after she received the lorazepam. The next morning, Mrs. Sanders was more alert, with pain now localized to her pelvis, buttocks, and perineum as before and with much less myoclonus. She was still very frightened and mistrustful, with persistent hallucinations. Her pain was now 15+/10.

Treatment of Delirium
and Opioid Equianalgesic Dosing

What is happening now? Mrs. Sanders has untreated delirium and inadequately treated pain. In a double-blind, randomized controlled trial, lorazepam was found to be ineffective in reversing delirium (Breitbart, Marotta, Platt, Weisman, Derevenco, et al., 1996). Delirium reversed only in response to antipsychotic agents (haloperidol, chlorpromazine) titrated to effect. Newer atypical agents (e.g., olanzapine) have shown efficacy in case studies, but haloperidol is the recommended initial agent unless there is a known hypersensitivity to it (Jackson & Lipman, 2005). Several days after Mrs. Sanders received a standing dose of haloperidol every six hours, along with extra doses for agitation (not to exceed 20 mg per day), her hallucinations disappeared entirely; over the next week, she regained her normal personality and was no longer fearful or distrustful.

In performing the opioid rotation, her medical team had miscalculated the equianalgesic dose of hydromorphone and consequently had undertreated her pain. Mrs. Sanders' pain had been at a 5/10 level before the exacerbation over the weekend. To achieve this, she had been taking 1500 mg of oral morphine. When she was admitted, therefore, she should have been started on a hydromorphone dose that was at least equivalent to that dose of oral morphine. But her 1 mg/hour hydromorphone drip was only 50% of the correct dose of hydromorphone; she needed a 2 mg/hour hydromorphone infusion.

How could the team have calculated the correct hydromorphone dose? First, calculate the equianalgesic dose of the total daily dose of intravenous hydromorphone. Because 30 mg of oral morphine equals 1.5 mg of intravenous or subcutaneous hydromorphone (Miaskowski et al., 2005) (chapter 5), 1500 mg of oral morphine per 24 hours is equivalent to 75 mg IV hydromorphone per 24 hours. But patients become tolerant to the respiratory depression and sedation that opioids induce. When a new opioid is begun, there is only partial tolerance to the new opioid. Giving a full equianalgesic dose can cause respiratory depression or sedation. Generally, therefore, the calculated equianalgesic dose of the new opioid is decreased by about one third. When patients have uncontrolled pain, the dose is not always decreased, but it was difficult to determine how much Mrs. Sanders' delirium was contributing to her pain rating (Coyle et al., 1994). To be conservative, we would decrease the 75 mg dose by one third (i.e., by 25 mg) and start the hydromorphone infusion at 50 mg per 24 hours, or about 2 mg/hour. We would offer bolus doses for breakthrough pain of 2.5 mg intravenously every two hours as needed. We would also consider adding intravenous dexamethasone if she had tolerated it in the past with her chemotherapy, but some clinicians would wait until she was less delirious to try this adjuvant.

METHADONE

Because using dexamethasone might be problematic, we might have used methadone to treat her pain syndrome. We could have used an IV drip or, if she could tolerate oral medications, oral methadone. Why methadone? Oral methadone is not only the most inexpensive agent for severe pain, its mechanism of action and anecdotal observation suggest that it has particular efficacy in patients with neuropathic pain (Bruera & Sweeney, 2002). Methadone is a combination of racemic isomers that not only bind opioid receptors but also bind N-methyl-D-aspartate (NMDA) receptors which, when activated, block the ability of opioids to inhibit the transmission of the pain signal from the periphery to the central nervous system. The greater the neuropathic injury, the higher the chronic opioid dose, the more NMDA receptors are created in the spinal cord. The more NMDA receptors, the more potent methadone is. Ratios of other opioids (expressed in morphine equivalents) to methadone vary with the chronic dose of opioid (Table 1).

TABLE 1.
MORPHINE: METHADONE RATIOS (ABRAHM, 2005)

Oral Morphine Equivalent (mg/24 h)	Morphine: Methadone Ratio
<100	4:1
101-300	8:1
301-600	10:1
601-800	12:1
801-1000	15:1
>1000	20:1

USE OF NEW MODALITIES

It is the very rare patient who cannot achieve satisfactory symptom relief using the pharmacologic and nonpharmacologic therapies described elsewhere in this volume. Psychostimulants (e.g., methylphenidate) can decrease opioid-related sedation and confusion; antiemetics or a change of opioid can control nausea. But hospice clinicians may need to consult with interventional radiologists, orthopedists, nuclear medicine specialists, or anesthesia pain specialists to find relief for the rare cancer patient who has persistent pain.

BONE PAIN

Cancer patients with metastatic bone lesions or patients with Paget's disease benefit from monthly infusions of bisphosphonates (e.g., zoledronic acid). These agents not only reverse hypercalcemia but also provide pain relief (Coleman, 2004). If patients receiving this therapy develop myoclonus or other symptoms of hypocalcemia, they are most likely vitamin D deficient and will need replacement. Calcitonin can also be helpful for patients with bone pain.

Patients with radicular symptoms from vertebral compression fractures or pathologic fractures may benefit from kyphoplasty or vertebroplasty. No large randomized trials have been conducted, but case studies support the efficacy of these procedures, in which methylmethacrylate is injected into the fractured vertebrae directly (vertebroplasty) or after balloon reexpansion of the bone (kyphoplasty) (Jensen & Kallmes, 2002).

Rare patients with cancer-related diffuse bone pain with adequate blood counts can be treated by nuclear medicine physicians with radiopharmaceuticals (e.g., Strontium, Samarium, Rhenium). Phase III trials have demonstrated the efficacy of each of these agents, which emit localized beta irradiation in areas of metastatic disease. Cytopenias limit their use, as many patients who would otherwise benefit from them have compromised bone marrow, either from radiation or from ongoing chemotherapy.

INTERVENTIONAL METHODS FOR NEUROPATHIC PAIN

Some patients have intractable neuropathic pain syndromes that even methadone and neuropathic adjuvants cannot control without excessive sedation. For these patients, we consult with our anesthesia pain colleagues. Mr. Salazar (whose story is a composite of many patient stories) posed such a challenge. He was a 45-year-old man with resected colon cancer that recurred in his lumbosacral plexus and L1-L2 vertebrae, with expansion into his epidural space but without compression of his spinal cord. The tumor could not be resected, and he could not receive further radiation. He had a burning sensation in the skin of his lower abdomen and, because of his lumbosacral plexus disease, he had severe neuropathic pain in his posterior thighs bilaterally. His doctors made numerous attempts to make clear to him his limited prognosis, but he refused to discuss what he would do "if time were short." He was married, with a 16-year-old son and a 6-year-old daughter. His wife felt as he did, going so far as to put a sign on his hospital room door saying, "No one with negative thoughts is welcome in here." They had told the children only that their father was in the hospital to have his pain relieved and then he could come home. His oncologist was going to consider experimental chemotherapy if we could get his pain controlled.

We had titrated his methadone, dexamethasone, and methylphenidate and added nortriptyline to sleep and lidoderm patches for his hyperalgesic lower abdomen, which helped; but he was still unable even to lie in bed without excessive sedation. We consulted the anesthesia pain service for other pain relief options. They reviewed his MRI and felt that he would benefit from medications (anesthetics, opioids, clonidine) delivered directly into the epidural or intrathecal space through a silastic catheter.

Neuraxial Drug Delivery

The choice of a neuraxial drug delivery system depends on a number of factors (Abrahm, 2005) (Table 2).

Table 2. Comparison of Intrathecal and Epidural Catheters for Pain Control

Intrathecal	Epidural
Duration needed: >3 months	Duration needed: 1-3 months
No home care needed	Maintained by family/home care company
Quicker onset, longer opioid action	Patient-controlled epidural analgesia available
10X more potent opioid action	More opioid-sparing anesthetic delivered
Increased incidence of meningitis	Increased incidence of fibrosis if used 3–6 months
~$10,000–$20,000 per pump	Home care costs ~ pump cost at 6 months

Mr. Salazar's life expectancy was three to six months, so a temporary catheter, which lasts only weeks, would not be helpful. He could receive medications through an intrathecal catheter connected to a totally implanted pump or through a tunneled epidural catheter connected to an implanted port. The port would be connected by a Huber needle to a portable pump containing the needed medications.

But a home care company would be needed to provide new cassettes and supply and support the portable (i.e., not implanted) pump, and Mr. Salazar's insurance would not pay for this. It would pay for the totally implanted pump and visits to an anesthesia pain clinic, where he would get refills every other week or monthly, depending on how much medication he needed. Our anesthesia pain colleagues therefore suggested an intrathecal pump. Mr. Salazar was, it turned out, very reluctant to accept the pump. For him, accepting the pump would mean that he had lost faith in the ability of the chemotherapy to cure his cancer. His oncologist convinced him that, on the contrary, the pump might make the chemotherapy possible.

The pump was placed with the catheter positioned above his area of vertebral metastatic disease and, after a week of titration, he achieved very satisfactory pain control with a combination of bupivicaine, hydromorphone, and clonidine infusion. We were able to halve his methadone dose and stop the steroids, the methylphenidate, and the lidoderm patches. He was discharged home alert, with acceptable pain control.

Over the next 3 months, he received the experimental therapy he had hoped for, but by the fourth month, it was no longer effective. His liver metastases grew, and his vertebral metastases now extended into his epidural space and caused cord compression. The intrathecal pump was becoming less and less effective because the epidural tumor prevented the medication from flowing down to the area of disease. Methadone was increased, and the steroids and methylphenidate were restarted, but sedation returned.

KETAMINE

With the collaboration of our anesthesia pain colleagues, we added an intravenous ketamine infusion, which allowed us to lower the methadone and lessen Mr. Salazar's sedation (Bell, Eccleston, & Kalso, 2003; Fitzgibbon & Viola, 2005). Initially, the mild dissociation produced by a drip rate of 5-9 mg/hour of this pure NMDA antagonist was not distressing, although he reported feeling as though he was "watching myself talk." But he required increasing doses of ketamine, and the psychological side effects became intolerable despite prophylactic antipsychotic medication (olanzapine) and lorazepam.

LOCAL ANESTHETIC INFUSIONS

We next tried a systemic infusion of lidocaine (1 mg/kg loading dose over 20 minutes followed by 1 mg/kg/hour infusion for 12 hours of an 8 mg/ml infusion), which can be used in the inpatient or home hospice setting

(Ferrini, 2000; Thomas et al., 2004). Unfortunately, the infusion was not effective, and we were considering palliative sedation. But before we did this, we asked our anesthesia pain colleagues to try again, and they produced a miracle. They decided to anesthetize the sciatic nerves directly. A block at the sciatic notch was not effective, so they placed bilateral peripheral sciatic nerve catheters in Mr. Salazar's by-now-paralyzed thighs and infused lidocaine directly.

We stopped the ketamine, and Mr. Salazar's delirium cleared and he had no pain in his legs. We explained to him and his family that we did not know how long the catheters would last (several days, we hoped) and that when they came out or were no longer effective, we would have to sedate him for his pain.

He finally understood that his time was short and that he might have only a few days to say his good-byes. But we were very lucky: The catheters, which were supposed to last for 3-4 days, lasted almost 2 weeks. During this time, he made extensive plans with his wife and gave his children individual final blessings and advice. Family and friends from all over the country flocked to see him. In his last days, as he weakened and the pain started to return, Mr. Salazar called in his doctors and nurses one by one to thank them and share his joy at his realization that he felt blessed and believed he would soon be safe in the arms of the Lord. He accepted sedation as his pain worsened. His death (a week after the sedation began) was a peaceful, pain-free one, and he was surrounded by his loved ones and caregivers.

SUMMARY

Palliative care and hospice clinicians now have an impressive array of techniques they can use to relieve the pain of their patients at the end of life, to enable them to complete the work they and their families must do, and to minimize the trauma experienced by the bereaved survivors (Block, 2001). In addition to their already expert communication skills, these clinicians can enhance the care they provide to patients with pain by becoming familiar with assessing patients with chronic pain; developing expertise in the use of opioids, adjuvants, and nonpharmacologic agents and techniques; and collaborating with colleagues with special skills.

While funding these interventions remains a challenge and the technology is clearly not the focus of care, hospice clinicians are not betraying the philosophy of hospice if they use it in situations in which it is the only means to an end we all desire: comfort for our patients and their bereaved families. ■

Janet L. Abrahm, MD, FACP, FAAHPM, is a hematologist/oncologist and palliative care specialist. She is an associate professor of medicine and anesthesia at Harvard Medical School and co-director of the Pain and Palliative Care Program and the Palliative Care Fellowship at the Dana Farber Cancer Institute and the Brigham and Women's Hospital. The program includes an inpatient and outpatient consult service and a pilot inpatient intensive palliative care unit at Brigham and Women's Hospital. Dr. Abrahm graduated from medical school at the University of California at San Francisco (UCSF) in 1973, completed her internship and residency at the Massachusetts General Hospital, and served as chief resident at Moffitt Hospital of UCSF. After completing a fellowship in hematology/ oncology at the Hospital of the University of Pennsylvania, she joined the university faculty in 1980 and worked there until December 2000. The second edition of her book, A Physician's Guide to Pain and Symptom Management in Cancer Patients, *was published in June 2005 by Johns Hopkins University Press.*

REFERENCES

Abrahm, J. L. (2005). *A physician's guide to pain and symptom management in cancer patients* (2nd ed.). Baltimore, MD: Johns Hopkins University Press.

Bell, R. F., Eccleston, C., & Kalso, E. (2003). Ketamine as adjuvant to opioids for cancer pain: A qualitative systematic review. *Journal of Pain and Symptom Management, 17*, 296-300.

Block, S. D. (2000). Assessing and managing depression in the terminally ill patient. *Annals of Internal Medicine, 132*, 209-218.

Block, S. D. (2001). Psychological considerations, growth and transcendence at the end of life. *Journal of the American Medical Association, 285*, 2898.

Breitbart, W., Marotta, R., Platt, M. M., Weisman H., Derevenco M., Grau C. et al. (1996). A double-blind trial of haloperidol, chlorpromazine, and lorazepam in the treatment of delirium in hospitalized AIDS patients. *American Journal of Psychiatry, 153*, 231.

Breitbart, W., Rosenfeld, B., Roth, A., Smith, M. J., Cohen, K., & Passik, S. (1997). The Memorial Delirium Assessment Scale. *Journal of Pain and Symptom Management, 13*, 128-137.

Bruera, E., & Sweeney, C. (2002). Methadone use in cancer patients with pain: A review. *Journal of Palliative Medicine, 5*, 127-138.

Cassell, E. (2004). *The nature of suffering and the goals of medicine* (2nd ed.), New York: Oxford University Press.

Coleman, R. E. (2004). Bisphosphonates: Clinical experience. *The Oncologist, 9*(Suppl. 4), 14-27.

Coyle, N., Breitbart, W., Weaver, S., & Portenoy, R. (1994). Delirium as a contributing factor to "crescendo pain": Three case reports. *Journal of Pain and Symptom Management, 9*, 44.

Ferrell, B. R., & Rhiner, M. (1991). High-tech comfort: Ethical issues in cancer pain management for the 1990s. *Journal of Clinical Ethics, 2*, 108-112.

Ferrini, R. (2000). Parenteral lidocaine for severe intractable pain in six hospice patients continued at home. *Journal of Palliative Medicine, 3*, 193-200.

Fitzgibbon, E. J., & Viola, R. (2005). Parenteral ketamine as an analgesic adjuvant for severe pain: Development and retrospective audit of a protocol for a palliative care unit. *Journal of Palliative Care, 8*, 49-57.

Indelicato, R. A., & Portenoy, R. K. (2002). Opioid rotation in the management of refractory cancer pain. *Journal of Clinical Oncology, 20*, 348.

Jackson, K. C., & Lipman, A. G. (2005). Drug therapy for delirium in terminally ill patients (Systematic review). Cochrane Pain, Palliative, and Supportive Care Group, Cochrane Database of Systematic Reviews, 3.

Jensen, M. E., & Kallmes, D. K. (2002). Percutaneous vertebroplasty in the treatment of malignant spinal disease. *Cancer Journal, 8*, 194-206.

Kabat-Zinn, J. (1990). *Full catastrophe living: Using the wisdom of your body and mind to face stress, pain and illness.* New York: Dell.

Lawlor, P. G., Gagnon, B., Mancini, I. L., Pereira, J. L., Hanson, J., Suarez-Almazor, M. E., & Bruera, E. D. (2000). Occurrence, causes and outcomes of delirium in patients with advanced cancer: A prospective study. *Archives of Internal Medicine, 160,* 786

Lussier, D., Huskey, A. G., & Portenoy, R. K. (2004). Adjuvant analgesics in cancer pain management. *The Oncologist, 9,* 571-591.

Miaskowski, C., Cleary, J., Burney, R., Coyne P., Finley R., Foster R., et al. (2005). *Guideline for the management of cancer pain in adults and children: APS clinical practice guidelines series* (No. 3). Glenview, IL: American Pain Society.

Ott, M. J. (January 2002). Yoga as a clinical intervention. *ADVANCE for Nurse Practitioners,* 81–83, 90.

Quigley, C. (2005). Opioid switching to improve pain relief and drug tolerability (Systematic review). Cochrane Pain, Palliative, and Supportive Care Group, Cochrane Database of Systematic Reviews, 3.

Singer, P. A., Martin, D. K., & Kelner, M. (1999). Quality end-of-life care: Patients' perspectives. *Journal of the American Medical Association, 281,* 163.

Thomas, J., Kronenberg, R., Cox, M. C., Naco G.G., Wallace, M., & von Gunten, C.F. (2004). Intravenous lidocaine relieves severe pain: Results of an inpatient hospice chart review. *Journal of Palliative Medicine, 7,* 660-667.

Weiger, W. A., Smith, M., Boon, H., Richardson, M. A., Kaptchuk, T. J., & Eisenberg, D. M. (2002). Advising patients who seek complementary and alternative medical therapies for cancer. *Annals of Internal Medicine, 137,* 889-903.

CHAPTER 10

Complementary and Alternative Therapies for Pain Management

Donna Kalauokalani

INTRODUCTION

"Pain is more than the hurt…. It means fatigue, weakness, weariness, weight loss…."

—Patient with advanced cancer

This quote expresses the devastation and desperation caused by cancer pain. More than a symptom, it seeps through all aspects of one's being. It is a personal experience that one hopes never to endure, and others cannot fully fathom the extent of one's suffering. The fear of pain is not to be underestimated in its effect on the patient's well-being or its influence on behavior—patients often characterize pain as the most feared consequence of cancer, even more than the apprehension associated with the cancer diagnosis or with impending death.

The number of people who endure cancer pain is alarmingly high. Nearly eight million Americans currently have cancer, and approximately one million new cancer diagnoses are made each year in the United States. At the time of diagnosis, about one in every two to three persons is experiencing pain symptoms. In the advanced stages of cancer, the odds of experiencing severe pain increase to three out of every four persons, with some estimates as high as 90% of those with metastatic disease.

Not surprisingly, in seeking relief from pain and suffering and restoration of hope, individuals with cancer frequently reach beyond conventional medicine's boundaries.

TERMINOLOGY

Complementary and alternative medicine (CAM) comprises diverse systems, therapies, and products that are not considered part of conventional care. CAM therapies have come to include not only traditional systems of care that have been practiced for thousands of years (e.g., traditional Chinese medicine) but also therapies or approaches that have been only recently introduced (e.g., alpha stimulation). Some organizations, such as the American Cancer Society, define "complementary" therapies as those that are administered along with conventional care and "alternative" therapies as those used instead of conventional care. In real life, however, the timing and circumstances surrounding the use of complementary and alternative therapies are far more variable and fluid, and such rigid definitions are not useful. Thus, the acronym CAM is frequently used to describe collective therapies not considered part of conventional medicine.

EPIDEMIOLOGY OF USE

The use of CAM therapies in the United States has grown steadily over the past 3 decades. In the landmark 1993 report by Eisenberg, Kessler, and others, nearly a third of the interviewed adults reported some use of CAM. If prayer was included among CAM therapies, the fraction rose to two thirds. The age group most likely to use CAM therapies was adults between the ages of 25 and 49 years. In a follow-up survey 7 years later, the proportion had increased by about 10%, and increases were reported in specific therapies, such as herbal medicine, massage, megavitamins, self-help groups, folk remedies, energy healing, and homeopathy (Eisenberg, Davis, Ettner, Appei, et al., 1998). Expenditures for CAM therapies are estimated to be in the range of $36 billion to $47 billion a year, and a third to a half of that amount is estimated to be paid out-of-pocket. To place this number in perspective, in 1997, the expenditures for CAM therapies were greater than all out-of-pocket fees for all hospitalizations; these costs approximated the total out-of-pocket fees paid for physician services in that year.

Various forces are driving the increasing use of CAM therapies. Market forces are undoubtedly at play; the explosion of information readily available via the Internet facilitates the search for alternative approaches; and the use of CAM therapies may satisfy people's desire to be more actively involved in their own care. Dissatisfaction with conventional care also has been suggested as a motivating force. This dissatisfaction seems to stem from a sense of inadequate treatment for chronic conditions and/or for the symptoms of such conditions (e.g., unrelenting pain). Whatever combinations of these factors are at play, patients with HIV, AIDS, and cancer have exceedingly high rates of CAM use.

Other reasons for using CAM therapies might relate to a person's ethnic background and the growing diversity of the U.S. population. For example, it is not unusual for an immigrant to continue to seek health care from the system of medicine practiced in the country of origin. Such continued reliance on forms of care not considered part of the mainstream in the United States may strengthen the traditions for the individuals and at the same time introduce new systems to the general public. Many CAM therapies represent modalities that are used in the context of a much broader system of care.

SYSTEMS OF CARE

Worldwide, there are numerous comprehensive systems of medicine. One system is Ayurveda, developed in India more than 5,000 years ago. Ayurveda emphasizes the body, mind, and spirit, and therapeutic goals established in this system of care are designed to restore natural harmony. To facilitate therapy, the doctor determines the patient's constitution—evaluating the body, mind, and spirit for deficiencies, blockages, and sources of imbalance. Recommended therapies to restore harmony may include instructions related to diet, exercise such as yoga, meditation, massage, and herbal tonics.

Similar traditional systems of care evolved in China and Japan as well. Traditional Chinese medicine (TCM) also emphasizes diagnostic assessment of the patient's constitution and uses diverse therapies that include physical interventions such as acupuncture and herbal remedies. Treatment recommendations are likely to include instructions for diet and exercise. In China, TCM providers practice in the same hospitals as conventional medicine practitioners. In Japan, Kampo is the traditional system; it relies heavily on herbal remedies and is practiced by many allopathic physicians. In an interesting model for integrating past and present approaches, Japan's national health insurance plan covers costs related to receiving both Kampo and allopathic treatments.

Although they differ in their protocols and traditions, certain general principles are common to all traditional systems of care. First, every human is viewed as a blend of body, mind, and emotion, and good health is defined as a state of emotional, mental, spiritual, and physical balance. Second, environmental and social factors are known to have an impact on physical and emotional health. Third, it is understood that the human body possesses a natural ability to heal itself. Appropriate nutrition and physical exercise and reliance on natural products such as herbs enhance this inherent ability. Traditional systems of care aim to treat the patient holistically, using the gentlest approach and avoiding dangerous or traumatic procedures.

CAM Therapies

Specific CAM therapies have been adopted from traditional systems of care without retaining the context of their delivery. For example, one can receive TCM-style acupuncture with no connection to any other aspects of TCM practice. It is not clear how removing therapies from their usual context of delivery affects efficacy. The context of care and the meanings attributed to illness and treatments can have a strong bearing on clinical outcome, regardless of the system of care. Thus, exploring one's motivation for care and expectations for treatment may facilitate clinical decision making in productive ways. The CAM therapies most commonly sought to address pain symptoms include spinal manipulation, massage, acupuncture, physical movement (e.g., tai chi, yoga), and meditation, as well as a host of botanical and nutritional supplements. Pain conditions commonly treated with CAM therapies include back and neck pain, joint pain or stiffness, headaches, gout, and fibromyalgia. In addition, CAM remedies are sought to address broader consequences of pain and suffering, such as functional impairments, nausea, anorexia, insomnia, depression, anxiety, and fatigue.

A multidisciplinary approach is recommended for patients with chronic pain, integrating the consideration and implementation of appropriate physical, psychological, and pharmacological treatments as appropriate. In this approach, CAM can be a valuable component. CAM providers often pay particular attention to lifestyle and environmental specifics that may be vital components of pain treatment but are often overlooked. This vital information includes, for example, exercise and sleep habits, nutrition, relationships, and environmental irritants and pollutants.

ACUPUNCTURE

Acupuncture has gained in popularity in the United States over the past several decades. In 1997 a National Institutes of Health (NIH) panel issued a consensus statement on the effectiveness of acupuncture. The panel found that although much research was inconclusive concerning the benefits of acupuncture, clinical studies revealed compelling evidence for acupuncture's effect on postoperative nausea, emesis, and pain. In 2001, a large clinical trial on acupuncture was undertaken in Washington State. Cherkin and others designed a three-way comparison among acupuncture, massage, and educational materials (the control group) in treating low back pain (Cherkin, Eisenberg, Sherman, Barlow, et al., 2001). Interestingly, the results of this trial demonstrated that acupuncture appeared to be less effective than massage in decreasing pain and improving function. Using the same trial data, Kalauokalani, Cherkin, Sherman, Koepsell, and Deyo (2001) showed that the patient's pretreatment expectations for benefit might have had a powerful influence on clinical outcome, regardless of the actual treatment received. For example, patients who had a higher expectation to benefit from acupuncture did better if they were randomized to receive acupuncture rather than massage. Conversely, patients who had a higher expectation to benefit from massage did better if they were assigned to receive massage. In general, more subjects in this study had high expectations to benefit from massage, which might explain why massage appeared to have a better treatment effect. These findings underscore the importance of understanding the patient's treatment expectations.

In simple terms, acupuncture is the insertion of a thin solid-bore needle into the body for therapeutic purposes. Both physicians and nonphysicians practice acupuncture. There are an estimated 10,000 acupuncturists in the United States, about a third of whom are physicians. Kalauokalani, Cherkin, and Sherman (2005) conducted a national sample survey of physician acupuncturists and compared their practices with those of nonphysician acupuncturists. Many styles of acupuncture are practiced in the United States, including TCM, French energetic, Japanese, Korean, uricular, and trigger point therapy. An interesting finding from the national physician acupuncture survey is that despite different styles and training, there are remarkable similarities in the points selected by physicians and nonphysicians to treat a certain problem, such as low back pain. The high correlation of selected points is shown in Figure 1. This convergence of point selection, despite the different philosophies and approaches, suggests underlying similarities in healing techniques that have evolved through the ages. This is an area worthy of further research.

The specific therapeutic mechanism underlying acupuncture's effect remains elusive, but it seems to be related to the muscle stimulation that occurs with placement of the needle (Gunn, 1996). The degree of stimulation can be modified with rotation, application of cold or heat (i.e., moxibustion), electricity, or injection of a solution (e.g., local anesthetic, saline). The injection of a solution requires changing from a thin solid-bore needle to a larger hollow-bore needle. Trigger point injections are commonly used to relieve muscle pain in western medicine (Simons, Travell, & Simons, 1999; Travell & Simons, 1983); the mechanisms of effect for acupuncture and trigger point injections may be similar. In fact, studies comparing the injection of substances with no injection ("dry needling") have shown that there is no clear advantage to injecting substances (Garvey, Marks, & Wiesel, 1989). When a needle is inserted into a muscle, a local muscle or neural reflex is triggered; this is postulated to induce a spinal modulatory system that leads to muscle relaxation. The end result is generally better range of motion, along with pain relief. Consistent with this theory, acupuncture is used for a range of

FIGURE 1. TOP 10 ACUPOINTS SELECTED BY PHYSICIAN ACUPUNCTURISTS TO TREAT CHRONIC LOW BACK PAIN

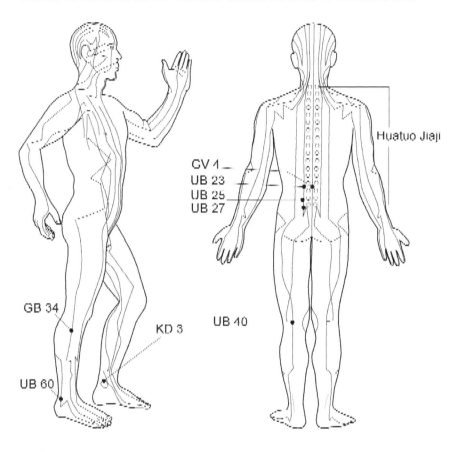

musculoskeletal ailments such as back pain, neck pain, osteoarthritis, and headaches. However, acupuncture is also successfully used for other ailments—including dental pain, asthma, nausea, and substance abuse (Spencer & Jacobs, 1999)—which suggests that other mechanisms are at play that are not yet well understood.

BODYWORK

The term "bodywork" refers to therapies such as massage, deep tissue manipulation, and energy balancing, which are used to reduce pain, soothe injured muscles, improve range of motion, stimulate blood and lymphatic circulation, and promote deep relaxation. Therapeutic use of touch is embedded in most systems of healing throughout human history and has been used for centuries to relieve the tensions of daily life. Many styles of bodywork are practiced today.

Chiropractic bodywork specifically focuses on the correction of structural and functional imbalances that stem from vertebral (spinal) subluxation. However, a high-velocity, low-amplitude thrust adjustment technique (the most common form of chiropractic manipulation) is contraindicated in certain anatomic areas as well as in the case of malignancies (Micozzi, 2001).

Despite the popularity of massage, it has received little research attention. The few recent studies on using massage for chronic low back pain show favorable results in terms of its effectiveness in improving functional outcome, reducing health care services, and relieving pain symptoms. Two additional benefits are that massage appears to be relatively safe and may be very cost-effective compared with other treatments for common ailments such as chronic low back pain.

Energy-based healing is one of the fastest growing CAM modalities in the United States. More than 67,000 health care professionals have been trained in Healing Touch (HT), and it is being used increasingly in clinical practice to treat a variety of conditions, including pain, anxiety, depression, and immunosuppression (Rexilius, Mundt, Erickson Megel, & Agrawal, 2002). Preliminary research by C. Cook and J. Guerrerio (personal communication, April 2003) supports the value of HT in reducing the side effects of radiation treatment, including fatigue, impaired physical functioning, and depressed mood. The differentiating features of HT compared with therapeutic touch (TT) are that HT uniquely incorporates several multicultural energy-based practices and has a specific program of study and an identifiable curriculum. Although several studies have documented the effectiveness of both HT and TT in reducing pain (Gordon, Merenstein, D'Amico, & Hudgens, 1998; Meehan, 1993; Post-White et al., 2003; Turner, Clark, Gauthier, & Williams, 1998), rigorous trials are still in the early stages of development. With the widespread use of HT, it is critical that rigorous clinical trials be conducted to evaluate its effectiveness in treating an ever-growing variety of medical problems. One of the fastest growing areas of HT use is in oncology. Hospitals throughout the country are beginning to hire HT practitioners to help manage the pain experienced by oncology patients and alleviate the distressing side effects of chemotherapy and radiation therapy.

One of the research design challenges in studying bodywork therapies is to control for the interaction that occurs between patient and provider. The intent is to separate the effects of actual touch from the effects of interacting with a caring human being. This distinction is important, as growing evidence in the medical literature points to the significance of the patient-physician relationship in determining clinical outcomes. In other words, the relationship itself is potentially therapeutic, apart from any treatments prescribed or performed. Notable healers in all systems of care seem to appreciate the importance of this relationship and the context of the clinical encounter. For example, Margaret Machado, famed Hawaiian *lomilomi* (massage) expert, when asked about the secret of her healing capabilities, replied, "If your hands are gentle, your mind is clear, your heart is loving, and you are present, your patient will feel the sincerity of your heart. His or her soul will reach out to yours, and the Great Spirit's healing will flow through you and bring a healing to both of you."

MIND-BODY THERAPIES

Release and relaxation, both physical and emotional, are common and important goals for treating pain symptoms (Spencer & Jacobs, 1999). Many CAM therapies fall under the rubric of mind-body therapies, focusing on the power of the person to mentally control physiological processes. These therapies are generally aimed at harnessing the body's innate ability to stop or reduce cycles of anxiety, other negative emotional consequences, and pain. Relaxation techniques include rhythmic breathing, progressive muscle relaxation, and meditation. Hypnotic techniques are also used to selectively focus one's attention to induce relaxation. Biofeedback uses monitoring instruments to provide physiologic information that can enhance one's efforts to induce a relaxation response. Training in attention and behavioral responses (cognitive-behavioral therapy) is known to have a favorable effect on managing pain symptoms. Self-engaging therapies such as yoga and tai chi combine principles of deliberate physical movement with meditation. Many mind-body therapies are so routinely employed in the context of multidisciplinary pain management that they are no longer appropriately considered CAM therapies.

Nutrition

Nutrition obviously affects the possibility of developing disease. Over time, a poor diet increases the odds of developing some type of degenerative disease, such as heart disease or cancer. The modern American diet has been criticized as being woefully inadequate to maintain optimal health. The food we eat affects the toxic free radicals in the body that are produced as a by-product of normal metabolism. Poor nutrition can heighten "oxidative stress"; conversely, nutrient-dense foods, such as fresh fruits and vegetables, provide antioxidants that reduce the free radical load and the resulting damage. CAM providers may recommend dietary modifications to restore nutritional balance.

Nutrition also can have a role in pain control. Proper nutrition may minimize pain and discomfort and ease the management of symptoms and side effects such as constipation. At the end of life, nutritional needs have to be balanced with the goal of enhancing patient comfort by offering familiar, favorite foods that enhance the final days for patients and their families.

Herbal Medicine

Herbal medicine uses plants or plant parts for their medicinal action. In general, herbal medicines act via their chemical makeup, just as conventional pharmaceuticals do. In fact, many plant compounds have been purified into pharmaceutical drugs; for example, digoxin (from foxglove), colchicine (from autumn crocus), and morphine (from the opium poppy) (Burton Goldberg Group, 1994). Nonpurified herbs and plants are generally slower and less dramatic in their effect than purified drugs administered by direct routes. With skillful selection, however, herbal medicines can facilitate healing for chronic problems. Caution is advised, though, as the common assumption that herbs act slowly and mildly is not necessarily true. Adverse effects can occur from a too-high dose, a low-quality herb, or the wrong herb.

Summary

CAM therapies, in their many and varied forms, are a valuable component of multidisciplinary pain care. The role these therapies play in health care and pain management is growing and evolving, and they are influencing how health care is delivered in the United States and other countries. The context of their delivery (including both provider and patient factors) is complex, and appropriate selection of therapies is not amenable to simple menus. A greater appreciation of these complexities is important to ongoing research that is attempting to elucidate the mechanisms, cost-effectiveness, and outcomes of various therapies. But even as research results unfold, CAM therapies will continue to play an important role in comforting, relieving, and relaxing people who are dealing with painful conditions at the end of life. ■

Donna Kalauokalani, MD, MPH, is director of health outcomes research at the University of California Davis, Division of Pain Medicine. Prior to joining UC-Davis, Dr. Kalauokalani was on the faculty of Washington University Pain Center in St. Louis. Dr. Kalauokalani received her medical degree from the University of Hawaii John A. Burns School of Medicine. She has completed postgraduate training in anesthesiology, pain medicine, preventive medicine, public health, and in health services research. She completed a prestigious fellowship in the Robert Wood Johnson Clinical Scholar's program and obtained her master's degree in public health at the University of Washington in Seattle. Currently, Dr. Kalauokalani's clinical interests focus upon health care for low back pain and the management of pains related to injuries of the nervous system. Her research interest focuses on factors that influence need, demand, and utilization of both conventional and alternative pain management services and how these factors affect clinical outcomes in therapeutic trials.

REFERENCES

Burton Goldberg Group. (1994). *Alternative medicine: The definitive guide.* Puyallup,WA: Future Medicine Publishing.

Cherkin, D. C., Eisenberg, D., Sherman, K. J., Barlow, W, Kaptchuk, T. J., Street, J., et al (2001). Randomized trial comparing traditional Chinese medical acupuncture, therapeutic massage, and self-care education for chronic low back pain. *Archives of Internal Medicine, 161*(8), 1081-1088.

Eisenberg, D. M., Davis, R. B., Ettner, S. L., Appei, S., Wilkey, S., & Van Rompay, M. (1998). Trends in alternative medicine use in the United States, 1990-1997: Results of a follow-up national survey. *Journal of the American Medical Association, 280*(18), 1569-1575.

Eisenberg, D. M., Kessler, R. C., Foster, C., Norlock, F. E., Calkins, D. R., & Delbanco, T. L. (1993). Unconventional medicine in the United States: Prevalence, costs, and patterns of use. *New England Journal of Medicine, 328*(4), 246-252.

Garvey, T. A., Marks, M. R., & Wiesel, S. W. (1989). A prospective, randomized, double-blind evaluation of trigger-point injection therapy for low-back pain. *Spine, 14*(9), 962-964.

Gordon, A., Merenstein, J. H., D'Amico, F., & Hudgens, D. (1998). The effects of therapeutic touch on patients with osteoarthritis of the knee. *Journal of Family Practice, 47*(4), 271-277.

Gunn, C. C. (1996). *The Gunn approach to the treatment of chronic pain: Intramuscularstimulation for myofascial pain of radiculopathic origin* (2nd ed.). New York: Churchill Livingstone.

Kalauokalani, D., Cherkin, D. C., Sherman, K. J., Koepsell, T. D., & Deyo, R. A. (2001). Lessons from a trial of acupuncture and massage for low back pain: Patient expectations and treatment effects. *Spine, 26*(13), 1418-1424.

Kalauokalani, D., Cherkin, D. C., & Sherman, K. J. (2005). A comparison of physician and nonphysician acupuncture treatment for chronic low back pain. *Clinical Journal of Pain, 21*(5), 406-411.

Meehan, T. C. (1993). Therapeutic touch and postoperative pain: A Rogerian research study. *Nursing Science Quarterly, 6*(2), 69-78.

Micozzi, M. S. (2001). *Fundamentals of complementary and alternative medicine* (2nd ed.). New York: Churchill Livingstone.

National Institutes of Health (NIH). (1995). *Alternative medicine: Expanding medical horizons: A report to the National Institutes of Health on alternative medical systems and practices in the United States* (NIH Publication Number 94-066). Washington, DC: U.S. Government Printing Office, Superintendent of Documents.

Post-White, J., Kinney, M. E., Savik, K., Gau, J. B., Wilcox, C., & Lerner, I. (2003). Therapeutic massage and healing touch improve symptoms in cancer. *Intergrative Cancer Therapies, 2*(4), 332-344.

Rexilius, S. J., Mundt, C., Erickson Megel, M., & Agrawal, S. (2002). Therapeutic effects of massage therapy and handling touch on caregivers of patients undergoing autologous hematopoietic stem cell transplant. *Oncology Nursing Forum, 29*(3), E35-44.

Simons, D. G., Travell, J. G., & Simons, L. S. (1999). *Travell & Simons' myofascial pain and dysfunction: The trigger point manual* (2nd ed.). Baltimore, MD: Williams & Wilkins.

Spencer, J. W., & Jacobs, J. J. (1999). *Complementary/alternative medicine: An evidence-based approach.* St. Louis, MO: Mosby.

Travell, J. G., & Simons, D. G. (1983). *Myofascial pain and dysfunction: The trigger point manual.* Baltimore, MD: Williams & Wilkins.

Turner, J. G., Clark, A. J., Gauthier, D. K., & Williams, M. (1998). The effect of therapeutic touch on pain and anxiety in burn patients. *Journal of Advances in Nursing, 28*(1), 10-20.

CHAPTER 11

The Hospice Approach to Pain Control

Samira K. Beckwith

HOSPICE AND PAIN CONTROL

During World War II, a nurse in England was horrified when she observed how hospital patients had to "earn their morphine" by exhibiting excruciating pain. The nurse was Cecily Saunders, and she was so moved by this undignified display that she began research that led to the modern hospice movement. To Saunders, effective pain management was the heart of hospice.

Saunders' work emphasized two basic points. The first was that pain was a uniquely individual and multidimensional experience. She viewed pain as not just a biological event but a multifaceted one, consisting of four interrelated components:

- Physical pain—commensurate with identifiable tissue damage.

- Emotional pain—sustained by psychological factors.

- Social pain—abnormal pain, probably caused by the dysfunction of the central nervous system and triggered by a feeling of isolation from friends and family.

- Spiritual pain—not attributable to identifiable organic or psychological processes.

Saunders' second point was that because each person's pain experience is unique and because pain itself is multidimensional, an array of disciplines is required to care for people at the end of life. Over time, her thinking has gained the support of others.

"Effective pain assessment and management involve an interdisciplinary approach to treat patients for physical, psychological, social, and spiritual symptoms" (Marx, 2005, p. 22).

Accurate assessment and frequent reassessment are the cornerstones of effective treatment for the terminally ill patient. To address total pain, the assessment should include a thorough history, including pain and psychosocial history; physical examination, including neurological examination; and review of radiographic studies (Reisfield, 2001).

In their assessment of an individual's pain, the professionals who make up the hospice interdisciplinary team (IDT) work closely together to recognize and address the nonbiologic as well as the biologic aspects of pain. As a result, for example, a music therapist's conversation with a patient may yield information of value to the nurse that may not have been noted otherwise.

The role of the hospice IDT in pain management is to ensure comfort and enable people to live their remaining days with dignity. Hospice professionals know that we cannot add days to a person's life but we can add quality to the days. That sentiment, stated in one way or another, is often expressed by hospice professionals, as it sums up their role of caring for the patient beyond the curative stage and of administering pain management in the earliest stages of the person's dying process.

The hospice team typically includes physicians, nurses, pharmacists, social workers, home health aides, specially trained volunteers, chaplains, homemakers, bereavement counselors, and massage, art, and music therapists, as well as other therapists as needed to relieve total pain and meet the needs of each patient and family. Each team member is crucial, and each has a unique role in the hospice setting and in pain management.

THE INTERDISCIPLINARY TEAM

The Nurse

According to Kathleen M. Foley, attending neurologist in the Pain and Palliative Care Service at Memorial Sloan-Kettering Cancer Center, "The one group of people who know best about pain management are nurses working in end-of-life care…The hospice nurse is the 'reservoir of expertise' in terms of understanding how to manage pain and how to utilize medications most effectively" (Foley, 2005).

Hospice nurses have described themselves as the first line of defense in patient and family care. At the same time, they are integral team players. In many ways, it is the nurse who sets the tone and direction of care for the physician, the chaplain, the social worker, the therapists, and others. Because nurses are often a primary source of care, families turn to them for answers. Nurses are often in a position to determine whether the patient is being properly medicated, because they are familiar with the individual and thus able to read the more subtle signs of pain, such as tension in facial muscles when the patient is turned in bed.

The effective hospice nurse can serve as an advocate for the patient to ensure safe and comfortable dying at home or in another acceptable environment, such as a hospice house. Regardless of the patient's goals, even if those goals are not typical, the hospice nurse remains supportive. For example, in one case, a young HIV patient lived on a mat on the floor of her apartment and had no family contact. Because this is how she wanted to die, the hospice nurse made sure she had extra visits from the team, particularly after hours, to help her take her medication.

The Physician

Of the more than 100,000 medical school faculty members in the United States, fewer than 100 specialize in palliative care (Open Society Institute, 2004). Because many physicians are not adequately trained in end-of-life pain management, the hospice physician is a rare exception: a doctor specializing in pain management. In the IDT environment, the physician has a great teaching opportunity—nurses, therapists, and other team members can all benefit from the doctor's expertise. At the same time, the physician is made aware of the management of spiritual and emotional pain, and how that contributes to the overall well-being of the person and ultimately leads to a safe and comfortable death and the best possible experience for the family.

The Pharmacist

The goal of the hospice pharmacist is to manage the patient's pain as expediently and efficiently as possible. In the context of hospice and palliative care, this is not simply a matter of delivering medications promptly; it involves developing new therapies and analgesic compounds, finding new uses for conventional medications, and using newer techniques.

Like the other members of the IDT, the hospice pharmacist is focused on caring for the individual and meeting his or her unique needs. Rather than simply filling a prescription, the pharmacist is a member of the team. Team members collaborate and dedicate time and thought to each patient to determine the most comfortable and efficient way of administering each drug. The pharmacist may help assess the best way to administer this medication to this patient. For example, there may be a need to avoid intramuscular injection because it can increase pain. Instead, the pharmacist may suggest a relatively painless subcutaneous infusion—a needle that is under the skin but not in the muscle or a vein. It was hospice pharmacists who developed gel therapy as means of delivering medicine to patients who were uncomfortable taking their medicines orally. The gel is massaged into the skin, adding the therapeutic element of touch and providing further comfort.

Hospice pharmacists may also have a role in developing effective management systems that allow health providers to continue to assess pain control and monitor the many medications that a patient may need. For example, Hope Hospice pharmacists oversee a unique medication management system that relies on both collaborative practice and an electronic database with evidence-based protocols. The system has been well received by physicians, because it saves time for everyone when patients' symptoms are better controlled. Hope Hospice found that 94% of physicians referring to Hope elect to use the collaborative practice system. It relies on evidence-based medication management algorithms carried out by a team of hospice nurses, pharmacists, and the patient's doctor. The physician approves the protocols and the nurse assesses the patient and passes that information to the pharmacist, who documents the assessment and prepares a plan. After follow-up outcomes tracking, the physician receives a fax that delineates the care plan.

This system of integrated technology and collaborative process was developed with excelleRx, Inc.; it enables professionals from various disciplines to participate in a patient's care and make informed decisions based on real-time information.

The pharmacist remains an active member of the IDT after the initial assessments have been made and medications prescribed. For example, one hospice patient was experiencing a high level of pain even with seemingly ample and appropriate analgesics. The nurse mentioned this to the pharmacist, who suggested different medications. The patient agreed to try new medications, and the nurse monitored the patient closely. By the next day, according to his wife, he was standing, eating, and happy for the first time in a long while. Because pain is such an individual experience, the pharmacist has to be ready to try various approaches to manage it.

The Music Therapist

When they complete the initial assessment of a patient, members of the core IDT (physician, nurse, social worker, and chaplain) may refer the patient to one of the team's expressive therapists, such as the music therapist. These team members may detect depression, agitation, or family friction, for which music therapy may be an appropriate intervention to enhance comfort or reduce conflict. Music therapists work with the other IDT members to assess and address pain. Typically, nurses and physicians identify referrals for physical pain, while social workers ask for help with the emotional pain of the patient or family members.

Many hospice patients are able to participate in expressive therapy with the assistance of music therapists. "Research in the area of pain management supports the effectiveness of music as a nonpharmacologic method of pain reduction by increasing levels of endorphins" (Halstead & Roscoe, 2002, p. 332). Music therapists attest to the power of music to help dying patients find validation of their lives through their memories and emotions.

Music therapy can also benefit the grieving survivor. The widow of a hospice patient (herself a former opera singer) was unable to find relief in bereavement counseling and was referred to the hospice music therapist. She began seeing the therapist every week, and they would sing and play music together. Eventually, she was able to talk and reminisce about her husband and her career. By the first anniversary of her husband's death, there was a noticeable and consistent upswing in the widow's mood.

The Art Therapist

Art is another form of expressive therapy that has been proven to benefit hospice patients and their families. Art therapy emphasizes the process of being creative and exploring one's emotions, and neither talent nor experience is a prerequisite. The patient's artwork—whether it be painting, drawing, sculpting; or creative or memoir writing—is not interpreted or evaluated. The act of creating can itself help the patient or family member achieve goals associated with pain management, such as decreasing anxiety or increasing relaxation. It can also provide an opportunity for life review and reminiscence, and an opportunity for family communication.

Art therapy is another opportunity for IDT members to support each other for the good of the patient: The nurse may recognize the need for the involvement of an art therapist, while the art therapist may observe a condition that should be brought to the attention of the nurse. In hospice, the team approach to pain control results in a continuum of care for the patient and family.

The Massage Therapist

Research is currently under way at the University of Colorado Health Sciences Center to determine whether moving touch therapy reduces the burden of symptoms of patients in advanced stages of cancer. Therapists at Hope Hospice (a participant in the study) have found that massage therapy satisfies the need for nurturing touch, increases the flow of oxygen to the tissue, and releases endorphins, the body's natural painkiller.

The massage therapist relies heavily on the other members of the IDT in assessment and intervention. At Hope Hospice, a massage therapist worked with a young woman diagnosed with ovarian cancer and lymph node involvement who had developed ascites (excess fluid in the peritoneal cavity), which caused abdominal and lower back pain. Having the fluid drained from her abdomen every 5 days was a source of great anxiety and fear, and the patient wanted a noninvasive way to control the fluid imbalances. Through nursing and massage therapy intervention, both the fluid imbalances and the anxiety were brought under control.

The Chaplain

For many patients, there is a spiritual dimension to pain; evidence exists to support spirituality as being helpful to many who are suffering persistently (Sundbloom, Haikonen, Niemi-Pynttari, & Tigerstedt, 1994).

Chaplains in hospice and other settings acknowledge that symptom control of physical pain often paves the way for spiritual healing. When the time seems right, the chaplain begins the work of helping the patient through such issues as finding meaning and self-worth, patching up family differences, and seeking forgiveness. Just as the patient's relief from physical pain can lead to spiritual pain relief, other members of the IDT know that progress in the spiritual area can help to ease physical and emotional suffering. The chaplain's assessment is a required agenda item in the weekly team meetings, morning reports, and in consultation with other team members.

The Social Worker

Patricia Prem, MSW, a member of the Project on Death in America advisory board, describes social workers as integral members of the interdisciplinary palliative care team who advocate for the patient and family (Open Society Institute, 2004).

Emotional pain can quickly spread through the entire family when a loved one is dying. Along with coming to terms with an impending death, many families must struggle with an uncertain financial future and other peripheral issues. The patient and family face changes they cannot control, which can result in feelings of helplessness, fear, and guilt. The social worker conducts an initial assessment to determine the family's understanding of the illness and its ramifications. Ideally, the social worker helps the family prevent a problem or concern from becoming a crisis. The social worker helps the patient understand and plan care goals and desired outcomes, and choose interventions to address pain. Patients may discuss concerns about the family they are leaving behind; these fears may increase anxiety and, therefore, exacerbate pain.

The social worker is constantly aware of the actions being taken by other IDT members to address the patient's needs, to ensure that all the actions are coordinated.

The Bereavement Counselor

The work of the other IDT members in the reduction of the patient's pain and suffering often reduces the impact of the family's grief. Counselors are usually needed to provide some level of support before the patient's death and, for the family, for a year or more after the patient's death.

Many hospices are particularly sensitive to the needs of children who suffer the loss of a loved one. For example, to help prevent children from carrying the trauma of personal loss into their adult lives, Hope Hospice annually conducts the Rainbow Trails Camp for bereaved children ages 6 to 16 at no cost to the families. The camp is open to youngsters who have experienced a death in the family during the past year due to any cause. Along with the traditional summer camp activities, the campers gain an understanding of the grief process, learn skills to cope with the pain of grief and loss, and learn how to say good-bye to their loved one. For the most part, the camp is a voluntary IDT activity—the bereavement counselors are joined by Hope Hospice nurses, therapists, and others who give their time to the children.

The Volunteer

The hospice volunteer can be a valuable adjunct to the IDT simply by being there with the patient when needed. In addition to companionship, volunteers may be called on for patient transportation and other team support roles. Trained volunteers can share their experience with the team, offering additional information about the patient that can assist in pain assessment.

Sometimes volunteers help in extraordinary ways, as in the case of the hospice volunteer who happened to be a dentist. A patient was looking forward to one last, happy moment in his life: a dinner with family and friends. Unfortunately, right before the event, his dentures disappeared. The volunteer came in immediately and worked all night to make a perfect set of teeth. He later explained that he could have made a set of dentures just good enough to get the man through the dinner, but he believed that the moment was too important. The volunteers take their roles as seriously as the professionals do.

TEAM INNOVATION

The very existence of the interdisciplinary team contributes to pain management. The IDT is not just a collection of individuals but a structure that supports the best collective decision making. The team is empowered to solve problems, even in very unconventional ways. The daughter of a hospice patient wanted her mother to attend her wedding, but the woman was unable to travel. Knowing that the mother had only a short time to live, the IDT orchestrated a complete formal wedding service in a matter of hours. The patient's bed was wheeled into the hospice chapel, where the hospice chaplain performed the ceremony.

COMMUNITY COLLABORATION

The IDT does not act in isolation. Hospices also collaborate and maintain relationships with others throughout the community, including hospitals, nursing homes, and assisted living facilities.

Total collaborative success lies in reaching beyond the medical community and into the community at large. Increasing interest in living wills and advance directives has given hospice representatives the opportunity to explain end-of-life care choices and related issues. By providing this kind of information, and articulating and demonstrating the hospice value of excellence in pain control, hospice helps alleviate people's fear that their loved one's pain and symptoms won't be controlled.

Comprehensive hospice care requires careful attention to the patient's and family's environment. Hope Hospice staff have had the experience of building three hospice houses in Lee County, Florida; with each new house came ideas for improvement that would add to the comfort of patients and their families. At Hope's new facility—Joanne's House at Hope Hospice in Bonita Springs—the walls are painted in soft, warm, textured earth tones. In each of the three patient care wings, the high, arched ceiling is sky blue and dotted with white clouds. The bubbling fountain in the center of the tiled floor completes the outdoor plaza effect, for patients who may be able to leave their care suites but can't go outdoors. Many of the 24 private care suites have a screened lanai on the back, overlooking a lake or a wooded area. The patient's bed can be rolled out on the porch. One patient actually spent his entire stay at the hospice house outside, in the warm Florida air. The 10-acre campus is ringed with aromatic walking paths. The offices and workplaces, although close to the patient suites, are hidden away to add to the effect of "being at home." For family members, there are living rooms, a library with computers, and a children's playroom, all in support of the goal of providing the most comfortable and pain-free experience possible for the patient and the family.

Regardless of the setting—whether it is a hospice house, the patient's own home, a hospital, nursing home, or assisted living facility—the hospice staff work to create a special culture: an environment of care and compassion to facilitate the management of pain and the reduction of suffering.

MEASURING SUCCESS

To measure and benchmark their effectiveness in pain assessment and management and overall care, many hospices use a survey known as the Family Evaluation of Hospice Care, developed and distributed by the National Hospice and Palliative Care Organization. The survey asks the family members about the care they and the patient received, and includes detailed questions about the effectiveness of pain and symptom control. Quarterly reports enable hospices to make comparisons with other hospices statewide and nationally. In the future, the National Hospice and Palliative Care Organization will provide a tool that will give voice to the patients themselves: a questionnaire to be administered soon after the patient is admitted to hospice care.

Independent studies such as the review of family perceptions of hospice by Baer and Hanson (2000) have reported favorable results. According to the respondents, quality of care for pain and other symptoms was good for 64% of the patients before hospice service; the percentage that received good care increased to 94% after the initiation of hospice care.

Through the modern hospice approach to pain control envisioned by Dame Cecily Saunders, patients no longer have to "earn their morphine" by abandoning their dignity. We have learned, and we continue to learn, how to recognize and evaluate pain and respond to it sooner rather than later. The mission of hospice is to provide exceptional care and support to all people who are touched by end-of-life issues, and the hospice approach to pain control makes it possible. ■

Samira K. Beckwith has 30 years' experience in professional health care and has served as president and CEO of Hope of Southwest Florida, Inc., since 1991. In 2004, she was elected to the position of national director of the National Hospice and Palliative Care Organization, the nonprofit membership organization representing hospice and palliative care programs in the United States. Ms. Beckwith is a frequent participant in national health policy forums and has provided expert testimony before government bodies, including the U.S. House Judiciary Committee. She has a fellow credential in pain management from the American Academy of Pain Management, the largest multidisciplinary society of pain management professionals. She is also a certified health care executive and a licensed certified social worker.

Under Ms. Beckwith's leadership, Hope has received numerous national awards for service and innovation, including the American Hospital Association's Circle of Life Award, the American Pharmacists Association Foundation's Pinnacle Award, and the National Hospice Organization's Heart of Hospice Award. In 2000, she was named one of Eckerd's Top 100 Women in the United States.

REFERENCES

Baer, W. M., & Hanson, L. C. (2000). Families' perception of the added value of hospice in the nursing home. *Journal of the American Geriatrics Society, 50*, 879-882. Cited by Marx, T. L. (2005). Partnering with hospice to improve pain management in the nursing home setting. *Journal of the American Osteopathic Association, 105*, 22-26.

Foley, K. M. (2005). Interview with Dr. Kathleen M. Foley. Retrieved August 16, 2005, from www.hospicefoundation.org/newsroom/ interviews/foley.asp.

Halstead, T. H., & Roscoe, S. T. (2002). Music an as intervention for oncology nurses. *Clinical Journal of Oncology Nursing, 6*, 332-336.

Marx, T. L. (2005). Partnering with hospice to improve pain management in the nursing home setting. *Journal of the American Osteopathic Association, 105*, 22-26.

Open Society Institute. (2004). Transforming the culture of dying: The project on death in America, October 1994-December 2003. www.soros.org/initiatives/pdia

Reisfield, G. (2001, May). Pain management at the end of life. *Jacksonville Medicine*, Retrieved July 7, 2005. www.dcmsonline.org/ jax-medicine/2001journals/may2001paincontrol.htm

Sundbloom, D. M., Haikonen, S., Niemi-Pynttari, J., & Tigerstedt, I. (1994). Effect of spiritual healing on chronic idiopathic pain: A medical and psychological study. *Clinical Journal of Pain, 10*, 296-302. Cited by Cavalieri, T. A., (2005, March). Management of pain in older adults. *Journal of the American Osteopathic Association, 105*, 12-17.

■ SECTION III ■

Pain Management and Control: Societal Issues

The issues of pain management and control do not affect only the individuals who are experiencing pain, but also their families, and the health practitioners who are involved in treating pain. Societal factors also deeply influence pain management. As discussed earlier, certain social attitudes inhibit pain management; for example, concerns about opioids and addiction may reduce an individual's or a family's willingness to accept such pharmaceutical treatments. This particular concern stretches beyond the family. Because opioid medications are highly regulated, physicians may be reluctant to prescribe them for fear of review and sanctions.

W.A. Drew Edmondson, attorney general of the State of Oklahoma, has been a leader in the National Association of Attorneys General. The association recently sponsored a series of listening conferences on end-of-life issues. One of the concerns that emerged clearly from these conferences was that every day people are experiencing pain that could be successfully treated. Edmondson notes the ways that state and federal policies may contribute to this problem. In his chapter, he describes in chilling detail how the Federal Drug Enforcement Administration (DEA), in response to a court case, in effect placed physicians on notice that a perceived high level of opioid prescriptions could trigger a DEA investigation and prosecution. Edmondson describes the efforts of the attorneys general to create a open dialogue with the DEA that will allow both state and federal policies to maintain an essential balance—empowering effective pain management while inhibiting the illegal diversion of opioids.

The "Beyond Theory" addition to this chapter offers an illustration of how federal and state drug policies can have untoward effects on patient care and arouse family concerns. A daughter expresses a concern that, after her mother died, the hospice staff whisked the medication away and destroyed it. "Was there an attempt to cover something up?" she wondered. William Lamers reassures her, explaining that such drugs represent a source for diversion and, therefore, must, by law, be destroyed. This vignette illustrates how even sound policies can touch the lives of patients and families in a negative way.

Timothy J. Keay discusses how these policies influence medical education—suppressing efforts toward palliative care and pain management. Keay focuses on medical education as he describes not only drug policy but also all the other factors that inhibit an effective emphasis on pain control in medical education. He notes that some of the most helpful current initiatives may shrivel up for lack of funding. Yet Keay remains hopeful that many of the new initiatives—an increased recognition of pain as the fifth vital sign, new curricula and resources, fellowships and research in palliative care—are signs that education in pain management is improving.

While Keay focuses on medical education, other educational efforts also offer reasons for optimism. Funded by the Robert Wood Johnson Foundation, Education in Palliative and End-of-Life Care (EPEC) is an ongoing educational effort designed to teach practicing physicians the basics of palliative care and pain management. Not only has the project been successful in reaching physicians, it has spawned a number of other educational efforts, including the End-of-Life Nursing Education Consortium (ELNEC), which offers a similar curriculum for nurses. In fact, EPEC has been a model for the Hospice Foundation of America's own efforts in clergy education (Abrams, Abbey, Crandall, Doka, & Harris, 2005).

Ben A. Rich, associate professor of bioethics at the University of California, continues this theme. Rich recounts the dilemma of the physician caught between an ethical responsibility to relieve pain and suffering and a regulatory climate that may sanction the physician who is too liberal in the prescription of opioids. While noting that medical education should include an emphasis on end-of-life ethics, Rich clarifies some of the ethical issues in physician-assisted suicide, total sedation, and terminal sedation that physicians and other health professionals encounter as they try to help patients manage pain at the end of life.

As always, the Hospice Foundation of America concludes its text with a list of resources. This is not just a helpful addition. It lies at the heart of hospice and the core of HFA's mission: to reassure dying persons, their families, and those who care for them that they need not face this final crisis alone. ▪

REFERENCE

Abrams, D., Abbey, S., Crandall, L., Doka, K., & Harris, R. (2005). "The Florida clergy End-of-Life Education Enhancement Project: A description and evaluation." *American Journal of Hospice and Palliative Medicine, 22*, 181-187.

CHAPTER 12

Policy Barriers to Pain Control

W. A. Drew Edmondson

State attorneys general (AGs) are not doctors; nor, for the most part, do they have a medical background. They do, however, represent consumers of medical care: They have responsibilities regarding abuse or neglect, and they ensure that consumers receive the "benefit of the bargain" and are not shortchanged when they purchase medical treatment.

In 2002 and 2003, the National Association of Attorneys General (NAAG) sponsored a series of listening conferences focusing on end-of-life care. State AGs were disturbed to learn that many of their constituents were suffering from pain that could be treated but was not. They were surprised to learn that over 40% of the residents of nursing homes in their states were in moderate to excruciating pain every day—and remained so 2 to 6 months after reporting it (Teno, Weitzen, Wetle, & Mor, 2001).

The listening conferences raised three consumer questions: (1) Will my wishes be known and honored? (2) Will my pain be managed? (3) Will I receive competent care? The answer to question number two was "probably not." Many reasons were cited for this gap in patient care, including fear of patient addiction, particularly if opioids were prescribed; insufficient medical education about pain management, which affects what doctors and hospitals do in practice; and the effects of state and federal public policy toward drugs.

While state AGs can have some impact on professional education, it is in the arena of public policy that attorneys general can make the biggest difference. As the chief legal officers for their states, they provide advice and counsel to state agencies, including medical licensure boards and law enforcement bureaus. They issue official opinions that—in most, if not all, states—have the effect of law, unless they are overturned by a court of competent jurisdiction. They can facilitate discussion between law enforcement and the medical community about the balance between effective pain management and the battle against diversion of prescription drugs.

LAW ENFORCEMENT

The state and federal governments have joint jurisdiction over narcotics in general and prescription drugs in particular. The same agencies that combat street dealing of prescription drugs and try to track those drugs to their sources also enforce the laws against cocaine, heroin, methamphetamine, marijuana, hashish, and ecstasy, to name a few.

The same agencies, if not the same agents, that raid marijuana fields, bust methamphetamine labs, interdict the importation of heroin, and engage in armed battles with street dealers are checking records in the offices of doctors who are registered with the Drug Enforcement Administration (DEA) to administer scheduled drugs by prescription. A doctor usually dreads the appearance of a narcotics agent.

Diversion is real. Drugs are sold on the street that should be available only by prescription, because they are dangerous when misused. These drugs are being abused and are causing damage to our society. Some are stolen from patients, sometimes by family members. Some are stolen from doctors' offices, pharmacies, factories, distributors, or supply trucks. Some are smuggled in from other countries. Some, unfortunately, come from doctors—doctors who grossly overprescribe, who may not even have seen the patient, and who are essentially selling drugs rather than providing care.

Pain is real, too. It can be described as chronic, acute, debilitating, sharp, dull, throbbing, excruciating, moderate, severe, intense, or exquisite; whatever its description, it is real. In proper patient care, it can and should be relieved. Overaggressive enforcement in combating diversion, without sensitivity to needs and perceptions within the medical community, hampers effective pain management by causing medical practitioners to alter treatment, which leads to inadequate pain management.

In October 2001, the DEA and 21 health organizations published a joint statement, "Promoting Pain Relief and Preventing Abuse of Pain Medications: A Critical Balancing Act" (DEA, 2001). The statement said, in part, "Preventing drug abuse is an important societal goal, but there is consensus, by law enforcement agencies, health care practitioners, and patient advocates alike, that it should not hinder patients' ability to receive the care they need and deserve." By participating in this statement, the DEA committed to an official policy of balance between combating diversion and appropriate pain management.

In March 2003, the NAAG followed suit. At its spring meeting in Washington, D.C., with only one dissent and one abstention, NAAG passed a resolution calling for a balanced approach to promoting pain relief and preventing abuse of pain medications (NAAG, 2003). The resolution stated, in part,

Now, therefore, be it resolved that the National Association of Attorneys General:

1. Endorses the joint statement from 21 health organizations and the Drug Enforcement Administration, "Promoting Pain Relief and Preventing Abuse of Pain Medications: A Critical Balancing Act."

2. Encourages states to ensure that any such programs or strategies implemented to reduce abuse of prescription pain medications are designed with attention to their potential impact on the legitimate use of prescription drugs. (NAAG, 2003)

At this point, the major players were on the same page. The administrator of the DEA was in agreement with the state AGs, and the state AGs could carry that message of balance to their drug agencies and local prosecutors. Egregious cases could still be prosecuted, but the prosecution would be accompanied by a restatement of the commitment to balance and an enunciation of why that particular case was worthy of criminal action. Borderline cases would be the province of state licensure boards, and aggressive pain management would be encouraged.

That train of good intentions was derailed in the fall of 2004.

Following the issuance of the joint statement on pain policy, the DEA published on its Web site a series of frequently asked questions (FAQs), with answers that were consistent with the new policy. The FAQs appropriately assured the medical community that factors such as the number of pain patients, number of prescriptions written, and dosages prescribed would not, by themselves, trigger a DEA investigation.

In the fall of 2004, however, the DEA was involved in the prosecution of Dr. William Hurwitz. That prosecution stemmed from an Organized Crime and Drug Enforcement Task Force investigation in Virginia that included the DEA, the Federal Bureau of Investigation (FBI), the Bureau of Alcohol, Tobacco, and Firearms (ATF), the Internal Revenue Service (IRS), the U.S. Attorney, and local police departments. During the trial, the defense sought to introduce into evidence the FAQs from the DEA Web site. The DEA removed the FAQs from the Web site, announced that they were inaccurate and incorrect as a matter of law, and issued an interim policy statement emphasizing that it could initiate an investigation based on just about anything. The court denied the defense motion to introduce the FAQs.

Lawyers can debate whether the court would have allowed the FAQs into evidence or whether, if introduced, they would have had any impact on the Hurwitz jury, which convicted the doctor on 50 counts of drug trafficking. A nonbinding statement of what might or might not trigger an investigation will not negate overwhelming evidence of guilt and would be, in the words of Perry Mason, "irrelevant and immaterial."

The withdrawal of the FAQs and the issuance of the interim policy statement, however, proved to be very relevant and very material to the delivery of health services. Members of the medical community perceived the move as a shift in DEA policy and believed that they could and would be investigated on the basis of the number of patients they treated for pain, the number of prescriptions they wrote for pain medication, and the dosages. Patient care was adversely affected.

On January 19, 2005, 30 state AGs and the attorneys general for the District of Columbia and Puerto Rico wrote a letter to DEA Administrator Karen P. Tandy (NAAG, 2005a). The letter referred to the 2001 joint consensus statement and the 2003 NAAG resolution, and to the fact that "both these documents reflected a consensus among law enforcement agencies, health care practitioners, and patient advocates that the prevention of drug abuse is an important societal goal that can and should be pursued without hindering proper patient care."

The letter continued,

> The "Frequently Asked Questions and Answers for Health Care
> Professionals and Law Enforcement Personnel" issued in 2004
> appeared to be consistent with these principles, so we were
> surprised when they were withdrawn. The Interim Policy State-
> ment, "Dispensing of Controlled Substances for the Treatment of
> Pain," which was published in the *Federal Register* on November
> 16, 2004, emphasizes enforcement and seems likely to have a
> chilling effect on physicians engaged in the legitimate practice of
> medicine. As attorneys general have worked to remove barriers
> to quality care for citizens of our states at the end of life, we have
> learned that adequate pain management is often difficult to
> obtain because many physicians fear investigations and enforce-
> ment actions if they prescribe adequate levels of opioids or have
> many patients with prescriptions for pain medications. We are
> working to address these concerns while ensuring that individu-
> als who do divert or abuse drugs are prosecuted. There are many
> nuances of the interactions of medical practice, end-of-life
> concerns, definitions of abuse and addiction, and enforcement
> considerations that make balance difficult in practice. But we
> believe this balance is very important to our citizens, who
> deserve the best pain relief available to alleviate suffering,
> particularly at the end of life. (NAAG, 2005a, p. 2)

The attorneys general requested a meeting with Tandy during their spring meeting in March, or as soon thereafter as possible; the meeting took place in April. In the meantime, the attorneys general responded to the DEA's request for comment in the *Federal Register*. Thirty-two AGs signed comments dated March 21, 2005, and made the following recommendations:

1. We urge DEA to clearly restate its commitment to the balance policy released in 2001 and commit to balance in all public communications. We also recommend that DEA consider appointing an Advisory Committee both to reassure all major groups (health care professionals, consumers, state and federal law enforcement officers) that are affected by DEA's actions and to assist DEA in translating balance policy into practice;

2. In commencing investigations, focus on factors that distinguish the criminal trafficking and diversion of pain medications from the legitimate and responsible practice of medicine and other health professions;

3. Develop a clear statement of policy that the preparation of multiple prescriptions on the same day with instructions to fill on different dates can be a legitimate practice;

4. Allow health care professionals to determine how to interpret communications by family members consistent with the requirements of their professions and licensing boards;

5. Develop an Advisory Committee or commission an Institute of Medicine study to consider in depth the medical, ethical, law enforcement, and policy issues involved in prescribing pain medications to former and current addicts for the treatment of pain and to report recommendations;

6. Consider the changing realities of health care and the patient population in the United States, in addition to changes in the nature of drug abuse, as policy regarding prescription pain medication is developed. (NAAG, 2005b, p. 2)

The comments of the attorneys general—as well as comments from the medical and law enforcement communities, consumers of health care, and others interested in this issue—are under consideration by the DEA in its effort to formulate a new policy statement. It is unknown at this writing whether the DEA will enlist the assistance of an advisory committee or work with the medical community in any other official manner.

On April 12, 2005, Tandy met with NAAG President Bill Sorrell and AGs Joe Curran of Maryland and Drew Edmondson of Oklahoma to discuss the states' concerns relative to the balance issue. On April 14, Hurwitz was sentenced, and Tandy took the opportunity to make the following comments at a press conference:

> DEA's enforcement strategy against doctors like Hurwitz hasn't changed. We employ a balanced approach that recognizes both the unquestioned need for responsible pain medication and the possibility, which today's case graphically illustrates, of criminal drug trafficking.

> To the million doctors who legitimately prescribe narcotics to relieve patients' pain and suffering, you have nothing to fear from Dr. Hurwitz's prosecution and no reason to refrain from providing your patients with pain medications when you deem it medically necessary. (Tandy, 2005a)

Tandy took the opportunity to reiterate that the DEA recognizes and appreciates the balance between the efforts against diversion and the promotion of effective pain management. She also assured doctors that the practices of Dr. Hurwitz were well out of the mainstream and that the appropriate treatment of patients' pain should not be affected.

On August 26, 2005, the DEA published in the Federal Register a clarification of its interim policy statement of January 18, 2005, pertaining to the writing of multiple, predated prescriptions ("Clarification of Existing Requirements," 2005). While still not green-lighting this practice (which many physicians use in the treatment of chronic pain), the clarification suggested ways that new prescriptions could be issued without forcing the patient to return to the doctor's office, a hardship for patients in rural areas and those with mobility limitations.

It remains to be seen whether the DEA's final policy statement will be dramatically different from its interim policy statement. The interim statement stressed what the agency could do as a matter of law: Under law, very little is required to initiate an investigation. If this fact is emphasized in the final statement, physicians will be "chilled" in their practice and patients will suffer.

Tandy could not meet with the AGs in March, because the dates of their meeting were the same as her presentation of budget materials to Congress. She made that presentation on March 16, 2005, and listed the agency's "remarkable achievements" over the past year as follows:

- collapsing Caribbean transit organizations that were moving at least 10 to 12 percent of the U.S. cocaine supply;

- maintaining dramatic reduction in the availability of LSD in this country through aggressive law enforcement;

- indicting 34 of the 42 current Consolidated Priority Organization Targets (CPOTs), the leaders of the most wanted international drug supply organizations;

- indicting nine and arresting four of Columbia's North Valley Cartel leadership who have been responsible for a third to a half of the cocaine brought into this country—two of the four individuals arrested are CPOTs;

- dramatically reducing the number of methamphetamine 'super labs' in America, forcing large-scale producers to retreat into Mexico;

- dismantling a Canadian-U.S. trafficking organization responsible for 15 percent of the U.S. ecstasy supply was a major contributing factor to a 10 percent decrease in the purity of MDMA pills (the lowest annual purity since 1996) and a corresponding 13 percent increase in price; and

- initiating more than 144 investigations involving the online sale of controlled substances without a prescription. (Tandy, 2005b, pp. 2-3)

These are admirable accomplishments and precisely what the DEA should be doing—things that state and local law enforcement do not have the resources or jurisdiction to do. But perhaps the DEA should defer to state and local law enforcement the regulation of their physicians. And, for the most part, state and local law enforcement should defer to medical licensure boards judgments regarding appropriate or inappropriate pain management.

MEDICAL LICENSURE BOARDS

Most doctors know that the odds are slim that they will become the subject of a DEA investigation, particularly an investigation that results in prosecution. Unless they are prescribing for pay without attention to a patient's overall medical condition and management or dealing drugs for profit, physicians would have far more concern that aggressive pain management, particularly involving the use of opioids, would come to the attention of the licensure board rather than of the DEA.

In 2003, the DEA prosecuted 50 doctors; in 2004, 42. However, approximately 350 disciplinary actions are taken against doctors by state licensure boards each year. For this and other reasons, doctors tend to practice conservatively, which can result in the undertreatment of pain. Two surveys that demonstrated this fact:

> A 1990 survey of oncologists studied the reasons for inadequate cancer pain management and found that 18% rated excessive regulation of analgesics as one of the top four barriers (Von Roenn, et al., 1993); a 1991 survey of Wisconsin physicians found that more than half would at least occasionally reduce dosage, quantity, or refills, or prescribe a drug in a lower schedule due to fear of regulatory scrutiny. (Weissman, Joranson, & Hopwood, 1991)

These surveys tell us what we intuitively know: If a doctor has two options and one is more likely to attract regulatory scrutiny, he or she will lean toward the safer option. That would be appropriate if the two options were equally efficacious and of equal benefit to the patient. But if the doctor's medical judgment says one thing and his or her sense of caution says another, then the patient will suffer needlessly.

In May 1998, the Federation of State Medical Boards of the United States (FSMB) adopted Model Guidelines for the Use of Controlled Substances for the Treatment of Pain (FSMB, 1998). This effort, supported in part by a Robert Wood Johnson grant, considered in a nationally organized manner the issue of effective pain management as it relates to standards of practice for medical professionals. The guidelines were submitted to state licensure boards for adoption in their regulation of professional conduct. The preamble to the suggested guidelines states:

The Board encourages physicians to view effective pain management as a part of quality medical practice for all patients with pain, acute or chronic, and it is especially important for patients who experience pain as a result of terminal illness. All physicians should become knowledgeable about effective methods of pain treatment as well as statutory requirements for prescribing controlled substances.

Inadequate pain control may result from physicians' lack of knowledge about pain management or an inadequate understanding of addiction. Fears of investigation or sanction by federal, state, and local regulatory agencies may also result in inappropriate or inadequate treatment of chronic pain patients. Accordingly, these guidelines have been developed to clarify the Board's position on pain control, specifically as related to the use of controlled substances, to alleviate physician uncertainty, and to encourage better pain management.

Physicians should not fear disciplinary action from the Board or other state regulatory or enforcement agencies for prescribing, dispensing, or administering controlled substances, including opioid analgesics, for a legitimate medical purpose and in the usual course of professional practice. (FSMB, 1998)

In light of the surveys described by Joranson and others, these statements, to be embodied in the codes of state licensure boards, were welcome words of assurance. Effective pain management was an appropriate part of medical practice, even if it involved opioid analgesics, and doctors should not fear regulatory action when engaging in such appropriate practice.

There was, however, a gap in the guidelines. Doctors could be sanctioned, even prosecuted, for inappropriate overtreatment of pain, but no similar opprobrium existed for the undertreatment of pain.

The FSMB went back to work and, in May 2004, adopted a new Model Policy for the Use of Controlled Substances for the Treatment of Pain, which was submitted to state boards (FSMB, 2004). Significantly, the preamble of the new model policy contained the following language:

For the purposes of this policy, the inappropriate treatment of
pain includes nontreatment, undertreatment, overtreatment,
and the continued use of ineffective treatments.

[T]he Board will consider the inappropriate treatment of pain
to be a departure from standards of practice and will investigate
such allegations, recognizing that some types of pain cannot
be completely relieved and taking into account whether the
treatment is appropriate for the diagnosis. (FSMB, 2004)

As of this writing, nine states have adopted the new model policy and
other states have it under review. If the optimal result is the appropriate,
effective treatment of pain, equal emphasis must be placed on overtreatment and undertreatment. Patients and their family members and
advocates must insist that pain be treated aggressively and licensure
boards must be made aware of instances where that does not happen.

Oklahoma adopted the 1998 guidelines and currently has the 2004
model policy under review. Additionally, in 1998, the Oklahoma legislature
addressed the issue of pain management as part of its code on controlled
and dangerous substances. (63 O.S. 2001, sec. 2-551(B)) The amendments
stated, in part:

The State of Oklahoma encourages physicians to view effective
pain management as a part of quality medical practice for all
patients with pain, acute or chronic. It is especially important
for patients who experience pain as a result of terminal illness.
(63 O.S. 2001, sec. 2-551(B))

If, in the judgment of the medical doctor or the doctor of osteopathic medicine, appropriate pain management warrants a high
dosage of controlled dangerous drugs and the benefit of the relief
expected outweighs the risk of the high dosage, the medical doctor
or doctor of osteopathic medicine may administer such a dosage,
even if its use may increase the risk of death, so long as it is not also
furnished for the purpose of causing, or the purpose of assisting in
causing, death for any reason and so long as it falls within policies,
guidelines and rules of the Oklahoma State Board of Medical
Licensure and Supervision or the Oklahoma State Board of
Osteopathic Examiners. (63 O.S. 2001, sec. 2-551(C))

And, most significantly:

The Oklahoma State Board of Medical Licensure and
Supervision and the Oklahoma State Board of Osteopathic
Examiners shall issue policies, guidelines or rules that ensure
that physicians who are engaged in the appropriate treatment
of pain are not subject to disciplinary action, and the Boards
shall consider policies and guidelines developed by national
organizations with expertise in pain medicine or in a medical
discipline for this purpose. (63 O.S. 2001, sec. 2-551(D))

In 1999, the Oklahoma State Board of Medical Licensure and
Supervision (OSBMLS) adopted rules pertaining to intractable pain,
perhaps in response to the 1998 legislative mandate (OSBMLS, 1999).
Those rules provide, in part:

To treat a patient's intractable pain, as long as the benefit
of the expected relief outweighs the risk, the physician may
prescribe or administer Schedule II, III, IV or V controlled
dangerous substances or other pain-relieving drugs in higher
than FDA recommended dosages when, in that physician's
judgment, the higher dosages are necessary to produce the
desired therapeutic effect.

Nothing in this section shall limit a physician's authority to
prescribe or administer prescription drug products beyond the
customary indications as noted in the manufacturer's package
insert for use in treating intractable pain, provided the drug is
recognized for treatment of intractable pain in standard reference compendia or medical literature. (OSBMLS, 1999)

Policy barriers to effective pain management exist at every level, from
the DEA to state licensure boards to local law enforcement. But with the
impetus of ever-improving medical knowledge and research, and the force
of public opinion, progress is being made, although sometimes with a
temporary step backwards.

CONCLUSION

At the conclusion of the NAAG project on end-of-life care, a report was published titled "Improving End-of-Life Care: The Role of Attorneys General" (NAAG, 2003). The section dealing with pain management was co-written by David Joranson and Richard Payne. Joranson, as noted above, is director of the Pain and Policy Studies Group, University of Wisconsin Comprehensive Cancer Center; Payne is chief of the Pain and Palliative Care Service, Memorial Sloan-Kettering Cancer Center in New York.

Their conclusion shall be mine:

> While affecting the life quality of millions of Americans, pain management is an issue that, until recently, has existed with little public notice or concern. Attorneys general are in a strategic position to ensure that residents of their state receive medical care that offers effective pain relief. The tools are now available. Health care providers need to learn them and feel safe in prescribing the dosage of narcotics necessary to relieve patients' pain. As states' chief legal officers who advise governors, legislatures, and executive agencies, Attorneys General can improve state policies, physician practices, and public knowledge regarding effective pain relief. As one state assistant attorney general described his motivation to pursue this goal, "When you ask yourself, 'What have I accomplished in my term?' You can say, 'I helped reduce the amount of human suffering in my state.'" (NAAG, 2003) ▪

W. A. Drew Edmondson is serving his third term as Attorney General for the State of Oklahoma. Before his election as Attorney General, Edmondson served three terms as Muskogee County District Attorney and one term in the Oklahoma Legislature. Edmondson is a Navy veteran with a tour of duty in Vietnam. Edmondson served as the 2002-2003 President of the National Association of Attorneys General (NAAG). Edmondson's presidential initiative during his NAAG term of office focused on examining the role of Attorneys General in improvement of care near the end of life. The selection of his presidential initiative was influenced by his wife, Linda, who worked as a hospital social worker for many years and served as director of the Oklahoma Association for Health Care Ethics and administrator of the Robert Wood Johnson grant to the Oklahoma Alliance for Better Care of the Dying. The cornerstone of Edmondson's initiative centered on three regional listening conferences which provided an opportunity for more than 50 attendees from Attorney General offices across the country to listen and learn about the barriers that prevent families from fulfilling the wishes of loved ones near the end of life. In 2004, Edmondson received the Dr. Nathan Davis Award from the American Medical Association, awarded annually to a statewide elected official for outstanding contributions in promoting the art and science of medicine and the betterment of the public health.

REFERENCES

Clarification of existing requirements under the controlled substances act for prescribing schedule II controlled substances. (August 26, 2005). *Federal Register*, Vol 7, No. 165, pp. 50408-50409.

Drug Enforcement Administration (DEA). (2001). Promoting pain relief and preventing abuse of pain medications: A critical balancing act. Joint statement of DEA and 21 health organizations. Retrieved November 12, 2005, from www.aacpi.org/regulatory/consensus.pdf

Federation of State Medical Boards of the United States (FSMB). (May, 1998). Model guidelines for the use of controlled substances for the treatment of pain. Euless, TX. Author.

FSMB. (2004). Model policy for the use of controlled substances for the treatment of pain. Retrieved November 12, 2005, from www.fsmb.org/pdf/2004_grpol_Controlled_Substances.pdf

National Association of Attorneys General (NAAG). (March 2003). Resolution calling for a balanced approach to promoting pain relief and preventing abuse of pain medications. Retrieved November 12, 2005, from www.naag.org/naag/resolutions/res-spr03-pain_med.php

NAAG. (January 19, 2005a). Letter to Karen P. Tandy, administrator, DEA. Retrieved November 12, 2005, from www.naag.org/news/pdf/so-20050119-prescription-pain-med.pdf

NAAG. (March 21, 2005b). State attorneys general comment on dispensing of controlled substances for the treatment of pain. Letter to Michelle Leonhart, deputy administrator, DEA. Retrieved November 12, 2005, from www.naag.org/issues/pdf/20050321-final-DEA-Comment.pdf

Oklahoma State Board of Medical Licensure and Supervision (OSBMLS). (1999). Oklahoma. Administrative Code 435:10-7-11.

63 Oklahoma Statutes(O.S.) 2001, sec. 2-551.

Tandy, K. P. (April 14, 2005a). Statement at DEA sentencing press conference. Retrieved November 12, 2005, from www.dea.gov/pubs/pressrel/pr041405b.html

Tandy, K. P. (March 16, 2005b). Statement of DEA administrator before the U.S. House of Representatives Committee on Appropriations, Subcommittee on the Departments of Science, State, Justice and Commerce. Retrieved November 12, 2005 from: http://appropriations.house.gov/_files/KarenTandyTestimony.pdf

Teno, J. M., Weitzen, S., Wetle, T., & Mor, V. (2001). Persistent pain in nursing home residents. *Journal of the American Medical Association, 285,* 2081.

Von Roenn, J. H., Cleeland, C. S., Gonin, R., Hatfield, A. K., & Pandya, K. J., et al. (1993). Physician attitudes and practices in cancer pain management. A survey of the Eastern Cooperative Oncology Group. *Annals of Internal Medicine 119,* 121-126.

Weissman, D. E., Joranson, D. J., Hopwood, M.B. (1991). Wisconsin physicians' knowledge and attitudes about opioid analgesic regulations. *Wisconsin Medical Journal, 90,* 671-675.

THE EFFECTS OF POLICY—A PERSONAL INQUIRY

Before my mother died, she was given morphine for pain relief. I am concerned that morphine hastened her death. In addition, one thing that my family noticed was that once my mother passed away, members of the hospice team were right there to throw out any morphine that was still in the house. Why so quick? Were they afraid someone else was going to take some of it and also die?

■　■　■

Morphine is an opioid and it is an excellent pain-relieving medication. When morphine or other opioids are used correctly to relieve pain they do not shorten the life the patient, in fact, many medical experts believe they could do the opposite by making the person feel better. Individuals who have a lot of pain during their final phase of illness usually die sooner, not later. Correctly used, morphine and other opioid analgesics are very safe, and they allow doctors to relieve pain and help achieve a comfortable death without shortening life.

The reason the hospice workers threw out the morphine after your mother died is because federal, state, and local laws require that they do so. Morphine is a controlled substance, and the law requires that it be properly accounted for. The morphine prescribed to relieve her pain cannot be given to anyone else. It is always destroyed in a regulated manner as it cannot be returned to a pharmacy. The law was developed to reduce the possibility that the morphine could be diverted to illegal use by other persons. The same procedure is used in every hospice program in the United States. Unfortunately, we do not always do a good job explaining these procedures to families, and unfamiliarity with the law enforcement requirements can cause concern, as it did in your situation.

CHAPTER 13

The Role of Medical Education in Promoting Good Pain Control at the End of Life

By Timothy J. Keay

INTRODUCTION

U.S. citizens' need for better pain management is not in doubt (Field & Cassell, 1997; Institute of Medicine, 2001). Multiple studies document the ongoing presence of pain throughout the population and the inadequate management of this pain despite the emergent need (Ducharme, 2005). For example, persistent pain is prevalent in at least 50% of older, community-dwelling adults and is poorly managed, even without adding the burden of a terminal illness (Weiner, 2002). Modern hospice to a large extent has been the leader in securing effective pain relief for people at the end of their lives, using medications and techniques that are effective in managing pain. However, hospice developed largely outside traditional academic institutions and is only now beginning to be incorporated into graduate and undergraduate medical training (Kaur, 2000). Effective training of medical students, residents, fellows, and practicing physicians in pain management is becoming more common and addresses one aspect of improving the ultimate desired outcome: effective and safe pain management for all patients.

The history of pain management training in American academic medicine has mirrored society's attitudes toward certain drugs, especially narcotics, and America's ethic regarding suffering. In the late 1800s, opiates were widely available in patent medicines, even from the Sears catalogue. With the rise of political power of the medical profession and, later, in the Prohibition era, the dangers of addiction were recognized and the use of this entire class of medications was marginalized. Thus, a medical textbook from 1940 could state, "Opium and its derivatives are usually taken in order to assure euphoria, or for the purpose of abolishing or escaping unpleasant reality. The more powerful the analgesic and euphoric effect, the more apt a drug is to cause addiction.... [Morphine] use rapidly creates a habit which is difficult to break" (Weiss, 1940, p. 607). These overstatements had no rational evidence base; more recent data suggest that addiction is much rarer, especially in cancer patients who have pain (Porter & Jick, 1980). In the "war on drugs," narcotic analgesics have become linked with suspect behavior, and the onus seems to be on the prescriber to prove in every case that it is correct to use an opiate. Prescribers who cannot prove that their actions are in accordance with the highest standards and guidelines of care may suffer dire consequences (Schmidt, 2005). At the same time, proper use of these medications has not been taught systematically nor encouraged by senior faculty, and has been neither well reimbursed nor considered consonant with ideal medical practice styles (Grossman & Sheidler, 1985). What physician wants to be perceived as running a drug mill, with a waiting room full of patients seeking narcotics (Weinstein, Laux, Thornby, Lorimore, Hill, et al., 2000a). Finally, it has been widely taught in medical education that pain is always a symptom of an underlying disorder, and good medical practice consists of diagnosing and relieving the underlying disorder, not masking the presentation with palliative interventions at the expense of delaying or missing diagnosis or treatment. For example, despite clear evidence that analgesic treatment of acute abdominal pain does not delay proper surgical diagnosis, there is a common reluctance to medicate patients until all physical examinations and laboratory or imaging studies have been performed and a plan of care formulated (Paauw, 1999; Thomas & Silen, 2003).

If pain management was taught at all, only acute pain relief with short-acting drugs, for a limited period of time, was advocated. Opiates were expected to be limited to dying patients (Weinstein, Laux, Thornby, Lorimore, Hill, et al., 1999). Thus, the professionalization process of medical training tended to reinforce negative attitudes and limit acquisition of knowledge of good pain management practices (Weinstein, et al., 2000b).

Progress is being made, however. Medical and surgical textbooks, curricula, guidelines, consensus statements, and teaching methods are being adapted to a more progressive and balanced point of view (Bloodworth, 2005). End-of-life care is an opportune time to improve the knowledge base, skills, and attitudes of health professionals toward effective pain control. Anesthesiology departments seem to be doing the bulk of education in American medical schools with regard to a basic knowledge of pain, but palliative care programs, geriatric medicine training, and general internal medicine and family medicine programs increasingly are providing needed skill and attitude training, as well as additional knowledge regarding pain management. Still, only 3% of U.S. medical schools require a separate course in pain management, while the remaining 97% include pain management as part (often not integrated into the overall curriculum) of some other coursework (Mitka, 2003). The first long-term evaluations of these efforts are just beginning to be published (Ross, Shpritz, Hull, Goloubeva, 2005). This means that progress is being made in medical education with regard to pain management, but that further progress and standardization of process and outcomes need to be pursued.

Nursing education has independently increased training in pain management and research (Sherman, Matzo, Coyne, Ferrell, and Penn, 2004; Twycross, 2002), as have other medical care providers. Accreditation organizations and even regulatory oversight are also helping to change the culture, so that pain management becomes a higher priority in the overall delivery of health care (Thomson, 2001). This chapter, however, will concentrate on the education of physicians in pain management.

GOALS OF PAIN MANAGEMENT EDUCATION

Medical education addresses at least three aspects of learning: knowledge, skills, and attitudes. These three areas of competence are essential enabling steps toward the goal of producing a practitioner who can provide patients with acceptable relief of pain with minimal side effects. Of course, the ability of the learner varies at different levels of training and specialization. A highly trained anesthesiologist with specialty certification in pain management should be able to manage highly complex pain disorders, while a recent medical school graduate would have a more basic ability. Thus, curricula, teaching methods, teachers, and teaching opportunities need to be tailored for the appropriate levels.

It is generally accepted that a new medical school graduate should have the knowledge, skills, and attitudes necessary to formulate a plan of care for treatment of common pain disorders, such as pain from metastatic cancer (Ross, Keay, Timmel, Alexander, Dignon, et al., 1999). This plan should include pain assessment, treatment, adjustment of medications, and management of common side effects. It may also include plans for referral to subspecialists for assistance in managing more complex syndromes. In Bloom's taxonomy of cognitive educational goals, such a learner should have sufficient knowledge and comprehension, and be able to use this knowledge and comprehension for basic pain control (Bloom, 1956). In contrast, a graduate of a geriatric fellowship training program might be expected to be able to assess, treat, and control a wider variety of pain syndromes with a wider variety of interventions and less reliance on other specialists. Such practitioners would also be expected to be able to analyze their own practice and effectiveness, organize and manage a pain management program, and be able to critically compare various methods or approaches to pain management, selecting the program(s) that best fit their population. In addition, a pain specialist would be expected to have such affective characteristics as acting consistently in the management of pain syndromes and being accountable for effective interventions, and would have adequate psychomotor skills to perform neuraxial blocks. Thus, curricular goals vary considerably depending on the level and type of expertise desired (Imrie, 1995).

Perhaps the most famous, widely studied, and widely applied pain curriculum is the three-step ladder of the World Health Organization (Stjernsward, 1988). This method of pain control and its associated educational program were designed for worldwide dissemination and implementation. It uses three levels of medication—aspirin, codeine, and morphine—in a sequential manner for increasing degrees of pain control, with or without adjuvant medication. This simple, straightforward, and easily understood curriculum is still the fundamental approach to pain management taught in all other curricula and has been proven effective by pain outcome research in tens of thousands of patients (Zech, Grond, Lynch, Hertel, & Lehmann, 1995). Obviously, this curriculum is not designed to teach complex syndrome management, nor does it directly address the skills, attitudes, teaching methods, local style differences, or incentives necessary for all situations. But it has been estimated to address the pain management needs of 90% of patients in pain.

More detailed curricula have been developed for pain management alone or for pain management as part of a general curriculum. For example, the International Association for the Study of Pain (IASP) has developed pain management curricula for medical, dental, nursing, occupational and physical therapy, pharmacy, and psychology professionals (IASP, 2005), and these curricula have been adapted for the undergraduate level (Watt-Watson Hunter, Penne-Father, Librach, Reman-Wilms, et al., 2004). Additional curricula have been developed that provide pain management education as part of a larger curricular goal, such as palliative care for undergraduate medical students, residents, or fellows (End of Life/Palliative Education Resource Center, 2005); geriatric care for residents, fellows, or practicing physicians (Education in Palliative and End-of-Life Care Project, 2005); and physiatry and rehabilitation medicine specialty training. Finally, curricula have been developed for practicing physicians, as is now required by the California Board of Physician Quality Assurance (American Medical Association, 2005).

METHODS

Despite the lofty goals espoused in many of the curricula, education interventions present many challenges in their implementation (Whitman, 1999). Methods of teaching that are appropriate and effective for the individual student must be developed, delivered, and paid for, and outcomes must be checked to ensure that the learners have the ability to provide effective pain management at the appropriate skill level (Lasch, Greenhill, Wilkes, Carr, & Lee, 2002; Ury, Reznich, & Weber, 2000). This is an ongoing effort in academic medicine.

For example, Sloan and others compared three educational methods for teaching cancer pain management to medical students and found that structured instruction on cancer pain management was significantly better than control or traditional instructional formats, especially when combined with home visits (Sloan, Plymale, La Fountain, Johnson, Snapp, et al., 2004). This study has yet to be reproduced in the education literature, although it promises to improve the ability of medical school graduates to manage common pain problems. Similarly, a variety of implantation techniques, drugs, and protocols are being taught to anesthesiology pain fellows in the United States, and there is a need for further research on the optimal curricula and methods of teaching for subspecialists in this area (Fanciullo, Rose, Lunt, Whalen, & Ross, 1999; Kopacz & Neal, 2002).

One promising approach to pain education is that taken by geriatric specialists. The need for pain education for geriatricians has been recognized (Weiner, 2002), and standards of care are widely accepted, including effective palliative care (Keay, Fredman, Taler, Datta, & Levenson, 1994; Luchi, Gammack, Varcisse, & Storey, 2003). Palliative care education is being routinely integrated into geriatric training for both residents and geriatric fellows (Montagnini, Varkey, & Duthie, 2004). This makes for graduates who are adequately educated in end-of-life care, including pain management (Pan, Carmody, Leipzig, Granier, Sullivan, et al., 2005). In addition, programs designed for nursing home physicians have been shown to improve end-of-life outcomes, including pain management outcomes (Keay, Alexander, McNally, Crusse, & Eger, 2003). It is, therefore, possible to incorporate pain management education for physicians with the ultimate result of improved pain outcomes for vulnerable patients.

RESOURCES

Publication of guidelines, textbooks, and other resources for pain management has proved to be generally ineffective in altering physician behavior (Bero, Grilli, Grimshaw, Harvey, Oxman, et al., 1998). While written resources have improved greatly in quality and availability over the past few decades, they cannot be expected by themselves to change the ability of medical professionals to provide effective pain management. Someone must engage the learner in the creative process of learning and ensure mastery of minimum standards of care. This is an ongoing issue in academic medicine, where resources are tightly controlled and subject to competing demands. The core group of faculty necessary to teach pain management has been slowly increasing, methods are in development, and higher standards are being required (Arnold, 2005). Yet it will probably be some time before good pain outcomes from American practitioners become the norm, as educational efforts continue and the patchwork system of medical care in the United States increasingly realigns its incentives and disincentives to provide such outcomes.

Medical examinations increasingly include more material on pain management; specialty credentialing boards require more training in this aspect of care, and licensing and regulatory organizations require higher standards of practice. These requirements influence the allocation of resources in medical education toward more attention to teaching effective pain management but do not directly contribute any funding. In the current university setting, it is not uncommon for only a small portion of the budget to be provided by student tuition or state educational dollars— monies that could be allocated toward pain management education. Reimbursement for clinical activities is not as high for pain management as for other high-tech subspecialty endeavors, and medical schools are increasingly dependent on research grants from federal and private sources. With the recent drastic and poorly publicized cuts in federal research dollars, medical schools and researchers are increasingly dependent on pharmaceutical companies for the basic support needed to keep the institutions viable. It is in the area of pain research that the education of future practitioners has the greatest potential benefits and risks (Washburn, 2005).

The National Institutes of Health (NIH) has announced interest in palliative care research, including, specifically, pain management research (NIH, 2005), but there is concern that the funding (if and when it is provided) will be too little, too late. Many universities have increasingly come to rely on private industry to fund new drug development or other marketable patents. While this provides a necessary infusion of funds that can then be used for educational purposes, it has a tendency to shortchange educational efforts (which are not the pharmaceutical companies' main concern), bias the education toward novel and as yet unproven technologies, and reward those who support an "industrial-education complex" approach to medical care rather than a more humanistic approach. It remains to be seen whether private industry is a viable model for educational support or only a passing fad.

In the meantime, it is important for medical education programs to systematically assess the resources available to them, their curricular goals and outcomes, the number and types of students, and the impacts of the interventions. Morzinski and Montagnini (2002) have described this process with regard to palliative care education for third-year internal medicine residents at the VA Medical Center in Milwaukee. Their logic model categories and process steps help explicitly define and assess the links between key components. This process also allows for a detailed assessment of the resources necessary to accomplish the desired educational results.

Perhaps with the anticipated recognition of palliative medicine as a subspecialty by the American Board of Physician Specialties (a step recently taken by the American Board of Internal Medicine and the American Board of Family Medicine), federal Medicare funding for palliative care fellowships will be forthcoming and can assist in the training of increased numbers of palliative care physicians and faculty. The successful funding of some junior faculty by K awards and MERIT rewards to do palliative care research is another welcome sign and a portent of better things to come.

OUTCOMES

The proof of educational effectiveness is in the care actually delivered and the outcomes that ensue. As previously noted, there is broad consensus that pain is not adequately managed in general and in a variety of end-of-life settings in particular. Partly, this situation results from inadequate education of health care practitioners, but this is not the only factor (Max, 1990). Other factors include low expectations by patients and organizations, regulatory barriers, and the costs of providing optimal care (Pargeon & Hailey, 1999).

The simplest way to ensure better outcomes is recurrent measurement of pain scores. Jones (1999) demonstrated that an educational program for emergency medicine residents resulted in improved patient pain scores. The Department of Veterans Affairs use and monitoring of pain as the fifth vital sign is a more global example of this approach (Geriatrics and Extended Care Strategic Healthcare Group, 2000). It may provide a quality assurance measure that pain relief is being provided. Unfortunately, it does not provide specific information on improving pain management that is absent and is subject to misreporting or even being ignored—a phenomenon all too commonly observed by practitioners in nursing home environments (Keay, 2003; Parmalee, 2004).

Other outcome measurements are also possible but need more study. For example, almost all hospice providers recognize the paradoxical phenomenon of prolonged survival once adequate pain control is supplied and overmedication and side effects are eliminated. Once patients at the end of life are more comfortable, they may not die as quickly as they would have without appropriate analgesia, despite the common myth that morphine hastens death (Von Gunten, 2005). With appropriate pain management, some patients may live longer, be able to deal with important end-of-life tasks, and even respond better to life-sustaining interventions. Thus, length of survival is not an appropriate measure of outcome at this time but requires further research.

One interesting approach to assessing outcomes of pain management is advocated by the University of Wisconsin's Pain and Policy Studies Group: Measure availability and use of opiates in various regions (University of Wisconsin Comprehensive Cancer Center, 2005). Although this is an oversimplification of the sophisticated approach used by these researchers, it is generally acknowledged that the cancer pain burden, for example, is approximately the same in similar population groups, so the cancer pain burden can be expected to be similar, implying that the use of opiates would be similar as well. What has been found, however, is that wide variations in the use of opiates exist from country to country and from region to region, even within a country or by different providers with similar patients.

A wide variety of pharmacy benefits management interventions also have been proposed, and sometimes effectively implemented, to improve pain management and physician performance (Stevenson, Pearlman, Green, Newland, Grondin, et al., 2004; Ury, Rahn, Tolentino, Pignotti, Yoon, et al., 2002). A complete review of this approach to outcome measures is beyond the scope of this chapter, although in the future, with the development of improved information technology modalities, this will be a fertile area for educational research. In summary, a multitude of patient outcomes can be measured and should be tied to evaluations of educational interventions when feasible.

CONCLUSION

Educational methods and efforts to teach pain management have improved and are being implemented more widely, giving hope that, at a minimum, educational barriers to effective pain management can be and are being overcome. Much more work remains, however, to ensure that the changes made to date continue, along with further improvements in pain management training. The final goal is acceptable, safe, and reliable relief of pain for all patients, with minimal side effects. ■

Timothy J. Keay, MD, MA-Theology, CAQGM, CMD, FAAFP, has taught medical ethics, geriatric medicine, and hospice and palliative care at the University of Maryland School of Medicine since 1988. He is currently Medical Director of Palliative Care for the Marlene and Stewart Greenebaum Cancer Center and the University of Maryland Medical Center in Baltimore, Maryland. Dr. Keay serves on the editorial boards of Family Medicine, the Journal of Palliative Medicine, and the Journal of the American Medical Directors Association.

REFERENCES

American Medical Association. (2005). *Pain management: Overview of management options.* Retrieved September 6, 2005, from www.ama-cmeonline.com/pain_mgmt/module02/index.htm.

Arnold, R. M. (2005). Mentoring the next generation: A critical task for palliative medicine. *Journal of Palliative Medicine, 8*, 696-698.

Bero, L. A., Grilli, R., Grimshaw, J. M., Harvey, E., Oxman, A.D., Thomson, M.A. (1998). On behalf of the Cochrane Effective Practice and Organisation of Care Review Group. Getting research findings into practice: Closing the gap between research and practice: An overview of systematic reviews of interventions to promote the implementation of research findings. *British Medical Journal, 317*, 465-468.

Bloodworth, D. (2005). Issues in opioid management: Review and analysis. *American Journal of Physical Medicine and Rehabilitation, 84*(Suppl), S42-S55.

Bloom, B. S. (Ed.). (1956). *Taxonomy of educational objectives: The classification of educational goals.* Handbook I. Cognitive domain. New York: David McKay Company, Inc.

Ducharme, J. (2005). The future of pain management in emergency medicine. *Emergency Medicine Clinics of North America, 23*, 467-475.

Education in Palliative and End-of-Life Care (EPEC) Project. (2005). Retrieved September 6, 2005, from www.epec.net

End of Life/Palliative Education Resource Center (curricula). (2005). Retrieved September 6, 2005, from www.eperc.mcw.edu

Fanciullo, G. J., Rose, R. J., Lunt , P. G., Whalen, P. K., & Ross, E. (1999).The state of implantable pain therapies in the United States: A nationwide survey of academic teaching programs. *Anesthesia and Analgesia, 88*, 1311-1316.

Field, M. J., & Cassell, C. K. (Eds.). (1997). *Approaching death: Improving care at the end of life.* Institute of Medicine Committee on Care at the End of Life. Washington, DC: National Academy Press.

Geriatrics and Extended Care Strategic Healthcare Group, National Pain Management Coordinating Committee. (2000). *Pain as the 5th vital sign toolkit.* Washington, D.C.: Veterans Health Administration.

Grossman, S. A., & Sheidler, V. R. (1985). Skills of medical students and house officers in prescribing narcotic medications. *Journal of Medical Education, 60*, 552-557.

Imrie, B. W. (1995). Assessment for learning: Quality and taxonomies. *Assessment and Evaluation in Higher Education Medicine, 20*, 175-189.

Institute of Medicine Committee on Quality of Healthcare in America. (2001). *Crossing the quality chasm: A new health system for the 21st century.* Washington, DC: National Academy Press.

International Association for the Study of Pain (curricula). (2005). Retrieved September 6, 2005, from www.iasp-pain.org/curropen.html.

Jones, J. B. (1999). Assessment of pain management skills in emergency medicine residents: The role of a pain education program. *Journal of Emergency Medicine, 17*, 349-354.

Kaur, J. S. (2000). Palliative care and hospice programs. *Mayo Clinic Proceedings, 75*, 181-184.

Keay, T. J. (2003). Back to basics in nursing home care. *Journal of Palliative Medicine, 6*, 5-6.

Keay, T. J., Alexander, C., McNally, K., Crusse, E., & Eger, R. (2003). Nursing home physician educational intervention improves end-of-life outcomes. *Journal of Palliative Medicine, 6*, 205-213.

Keay, T. J., Fredman, L., Taler, G. A., Datta, S., & Levenson, S. A. (1994). Indicators of quality medical care for the terminally ill in nursing homes. *Journal of the American Geriatrics Society, 42*, 853-860.

Kopacz, D. J., & Neal, J. M. (2002). Regional anesthesia and pain medicine: Residency training—the year 2000. *Regional Anesthesia and Pain Medicine, 27*, 9-14.

Lasch, K., Greenhill, A., Wilkes, G., Carr, D., Lee, M., & Blanchard, R. (2002). Why study pain? A qualitative analysis of medical and nursing faculty and students' knowledge of and attitudes to cancer pain management. *Journal of Palliative Medicine, 5*, 57-71.

Luchi, R. J., Gammack, J. K., Varcisse, V. J., & Storey, C. P. (2003). Standards of care in geriatric practice. *Annual Review of Medicine, 54*, 185-196.

Max, M. (1990). Improving outcomes of analgesic treatment: Is education enough? *Annals of Internal Medicine, 113*, 885-889.

Merrill, J. M., Hill, C. S., Laux, L. M., Lorimor, R. I., Thornby, J. I., Thorpe, D., et al. (1999). Measuring medical students' reluctance to prescribe opioids for cancer pain. *Psychological Reports, 84,* 28-30.

Mitka, M. (2003). "Virtual textbook" on pain released. *Journal of the American Medical Association, 290,* 2395.

Montagnini, M., Varkey, B., & Duthie, E. (2004). Palliative care education integrated into a geriatrics rotation for resident physicians. *Journal of Palliative Medicine, 7,* 652-659.

Morzinski, J. A., & Montagnini, M. L. (2002). Logic modeling: A tool for improving educational programs. *Journal of Palliative Medicine, 5,* 566-570.

National Institutes of Health, State-of-the-Science Conference Statement. Final Statement, Improving End-of-Life Care. February 18, 2005. Retrieved September 6, 2005, from http://consensus.nih.gov/ PREVIOUSSTATEMENTS.htm#EndOfLifeCare.

Paauw, D. S. (1999). Did we learn evidence-based medicine in medical school? Some common medical mythology. *Journal of the American Board of Family Practce, 12,* 143-149.

Pan, C. X., Carmody, S., Leipzig, R. M., Granieri, E., Sullivan, A., Block, S.D., et al (2005). There is hope for the future: National survey results reveal that geriatric medicine fellows are well-educated in end-of-life care. *Journal of the American Geriatrics Society, 53,* 705-710.

Pargeon, K. L., & Hailey, B. J. (1999). Barriers to effective cancer pain management: A review of the literature. *Journal of Pain and Symptom Management, 18,* 358-368.

Parmalee, P. A. (2004). Quality improvements in nursing homes: Elephants in the room. *Journal of the American Geriatrics Society, 52,* 2138-2140.

Porter, J., & Jick, H. (1980). Addiction rare in patients treated with narcotics. *New England Journal of Medicine, 302,* 123.

Ross, D. D., Keay, T. J., Timmel , D., Alexander, C., Dignon, C., O'Mara, A., et al. (1999). Required training in hospice and palliative care at the University of Maryland School of Medicine. *Journal of Cancer Education, 14,* 132-136.

Ross, D. D., Shpritz, D., Hull, M. M., & Goloubeva, O. (2005). Long-term evaluation of required coursework in palliative and end-of-life care for medical students. *Journal of Palliative Medicine 8*(5), 962-974.

Schmidt, C. (2005). Experts worry about chilling effect of federal regulations on treating pain. *Journal of the National Cancer Institute, 97,* 544-545.

Sherman, D. W., Matzo, M. L., Coyne, P., Ferrell, B. R., & Penn, B. K. (2004). Teaching symptom management in end-of-life care. *Journal of Nursing Staff Development, 20,* 103-115.

Sloan, P. A., Plymale, M., LaFountain, P., Johnson, M., Snapp, J., & Sloan, D. A. (2004). Equipping medical students to manage cancer pain: A comparison of three educational methods. *Journal of Pain and Symptom Management, 27,* 333-342.

Stevenson, J. G., Pearlman, M., Green, C. R., , C.R., Newland, S., Grondin, L., Thompson, M., et al. (2004). Altering meperidine prescribing patterns in a university teaching hospital. *Joint Commission Journal of Quality and Safety, 30,* 277-281.

Stjernsward, J. (1988). WHO cancer pain relief programme. *Cancer Surveys, 7,* 195-208.

Thomas, S. H., & Silen, W. (2003). Effect on diagnostic efficiency of analgesia for undifferentiated abdominal pain. *British Journal of Surgery, 90,* 5-9.

Thomson, H. (2001). A new law to improve pain management and end-of-life care: Learning how to treat patients in pain and near death must become a priority. *Western Journal of Medicine, 174,* 161-162.

Twycross, A. (2002). Educating nurses about pain management: The way forward. *Journal of Clinical Nursing, 11,* 705-714.

University of Wisconsin Comprehensive Cancer Center, Pain and Policy Studies Group. (2005). Retrieved September 7, 2005, from www.medsch.wisc.edu/painpolicy.

Ury, W. A. S., Rahn, M., Tolentino, V., Pignotti, M. G., Yoon, J., McKegney, P., et al. (2002). Can a pain management and palliative care curriculum improve the opioid prescribing practices of medical residents? *Journal of General Internal Medicine, 17,* 625-631.

Ury, W. A., Reznich, C. B., & Weber, C. M. (2000) A needs assessment for a palliative care curriculum. *Journal of Pain and Symptom Management, 20,* 408-416.

Von Gunten, C. (2005). Fast fact and concept #008: Morphine and hastened death. Retrieved September 6, 2005, from www.eperc.mcw.edu/fastFact/ff_008.htm.

Washburn, J. (2005). *University, Inc.: The corporate corruption of American higher education.* New York: Persus Books.

Watt-Watson, J., Hunter, J., Pennefather, P., Librach, L., Reman-Wilms, L., Scheiber, M., et al. (2004). An integrated undergraduate pain curriculum, based on IASP curricula, for six health science faculties. *Pain, 110,* 140-148.

Weiner, D. K. (2002). Improving pain management for older adults: An urgent agenda for the educator, investigator, and practitioner. *Pain, 97,* 1-4.

Weinstein, S. M., Laux, L. F., Thornby, J. I., Lorimore, R.J., Hill, C.S. Jr., Thorpe, D. M., et al. (2000a). Medical students' attitudes toward pain and the use of opioid analgesics: Implications for changing medical school curriculum. *Southern Medical Journal, 93,* 472-478.

Weinstein, S. M., Laux, L. F., Thornby, J. I., Lorimore, R.J., Hill, C.S. Jr., Thorpe, D. M. et al. (2000b). Physicians' attitudes toward pain and the use of opioid analgesics: Results of a survey from the Texas cancer pain initiative. *Southern Medical Journal, 93,* 479-487.

Weiss, S. (1940). Acute and chronic opium intoxications. In R. L. Cecil (Ed.), *Cecil textbook of medicine* (pp. 606-610). Philadelphia: W.B. Saunders Co.

Whitman, N. A. (1999). *There is no gene for good teaching: A handbook on lecturing for medical teachers.* Salt Lake City: University of Utah.

Zech, D. F. J., Grond, S., Lynch, J. Hertel, D., & Lehmann, K. A. (1995). Validation of World Health Organization guidelines for cancer pain relief; A ten-year prospective study. *Pain, 63,* 65-76.

■ CHAPTER 14 ■

The Ethical Dimensions of Pain and Suffering

By Ben A. Rich

INTRODUCTION

Pain management in contemporary American health care is a persistent and perennial problem. What distinguishes the contemporary problem from the one of 25–30 years ago is that it has, to a significant degree, become open and notorious rather than perceived and acknowledged by only a small cadre of pain and palliative care specialists. A host of reports and initiatives, particularly in the 1990s, moved significantly beyond previous efforts to deny or minimize the extent of the problem, and instead initiated remedial measures. Another phenomenon of this crucial decade was the widespread recognition that the failure of health care professionals to relieve pain and suffering constituted more than simply a manifestation of deficiencies in professional knowledge and skills associated with the assessment and management of pain. While there was certainly compelling evidence of the need for a major national undertaking in remedial education of health care professionals in the assessment and management of pain, there was also the acknowledgment—at least among a few of the more progressive opinion leaders in the health professions—that "to allow a patient to experience unbearable pain or suffering is unethical medical practice" (Wanzer, Federman, Adelstein, Cassel, Cassem, et al., 1989).

THE TRANSVALUATION OF VALUES

If one reaches far back into the history of the health professions, and medicine in particular, the moral and professional obligation to relieve pain and suffering, particularly (as was often the case throughout most of history) when curative measures were either unavailable or ineffective, was preeminent. Somehow, with the rise of the curative model of medicine and the rapid advances of medical science and technology, most notably in the last half of the 20th century, palliative measures became the last resort, used only when, as the process of dying became manifest, medicine was found "to have nothing more to offer." The prevailing view could be stated this way: Either ethics is irrelevant to issues of pain management and palliative care, or the ethical principles of beneficence and nonmaleficence require that health professionals be extremely conservative in the use of opioid analgesics because of the many risks and adverse consequences associated with their use in high dosages or over prolonged periods. This approach to the relief of pain and suffering greatly exaggerated the risks of opioids and unreasonably minimized the harm to patients caused by undertreated pain. But, more fundamentally, it sought to justify a remarkable and disturbing alienation of the medical profession from one of its core values: the duty to relieve suffering (Melzack, 1990).

LITIGATING THE RIGHT TO PAIN RELIEF

David Morris, in his seminal book *The Culture of Pain*, reflected on the profound failure of the health professions in general, and medicine in particular, to manifest any awareness of the moral dimension of undertreated pain. He theorized in the following grim terms:

> The ethics of pain management, unfortunately, may not receive proper attention until the first doctor is successfully sued for failing to provide adequate relief. At that point, the need for a full and reflective dialogue on ethical questions about pain will be preempted—as so often happens in American life—in favor of the slowly grinding mills of the law. (Morris, 1991, p. 192)

Morris proved to be remarkably prescient, for in the year his book was published, a jury in North Carolina became the first in the nation to hold a health care institution and professional liable for failure to properly manage the pain of a dying patient (*Estate of Henry James v. Hillhaven Corporation*, 1991). The nexus between law and ethics in the domain of pain management is exquisitely captured in the James case, and for this reason we should consider it in some detail. Henry James was a 75-year-old man with stage III adenocarcenoma of the prostate with metastases to the lumbar sacral spine and left femur. He had been hospitalized in a community hospital for complications from the disease, and during that time was placed on a pain management regimen that proved effective in controlling his pain. He was then discharged to a skilled nursing facility (SNF) owned and operated by the Hillhaven Corporation. The expectation of the hospital staff and his family was that the pain management regimen would continue.

Contrary to that expectation, and without any recorded consultation with the physicians who had developed the pain management plan, a senior nurse at the SNF concluded that James either was addicted or was at serious risk of becoming addicted to morphine. Without informed consent on the part of James or his family, she elected to wean him from the morphine and substitute a mild tranquilizer. The slightly over 3 weeks James spent in the SNF were chiefly characterized by uncontrolled pain. Following his death, his family filed suit against Hillhaven, alleging that he had been subjected to substantial unnecessary suffering in contravention of the applicable standard of care.

The plaintiffs' attorney called on expert witnesses from the National Institutes of Health to testify to the standard of care for the management of cancer pain. The nurse who had discontinued the opioid analgesia testified, "I have never heard of giving such high doses [of morphine] at such frequent intervals, or awakening a patient to give medication. I have seen patients much sicker and in more pain [than James] on less medication. The staff and I did not think he needed that much morphine" (Cushing, 1992, p. 23). The jury was required to answer these three questions: (1) Is there a recognized standard of care for the management of pain for patients such as Henry James? (2) If so, was that standard of care breached by the defendant in this case? (3) If so, what are several weeks of unnecessary pain and suffering worth in monetary damages? The jury answered the questions as follows: (1) Yes; (2) Yes; (3) $7.5 million.

The jury was not finished, however, and it is at this point that we enter fully into the moral dimension of the case. The law considers juries to be the conscience of the community; in appropriate cases, they may express moral outrage on the part of the community by awarding punitive as well as compensatory damages. Punitive damages are not intended to compensate the injured party in the litigation but rather to send a message to others in similar circumstances. The message when punitive damages are awarded is not to engage in acts or omissions similar to those of the defendant, for such conduct is deemed morally reprehensible. The jury assessed another $7.5 million in punitive damages against the Hillhaven Corporation, ostensibly in the hope that future patients would not be subjected to unnecessary pain and suffering at the hands of opiophobic nurses.

Ten years after the *James* verdict, the first physician was, in the words of David Morris, "successfully sued for failing to provide adequate relief." A California physician was found to have perpetrated elder abuse on an 85-year-old man by failing to provide adequate pain relief during a 5-day hospitalization that preceded the patient's death in home hospice. The jury initially awarded $1.5 million in compensatory damages and came within one vote of awarding punitive damages (*Bergman v. Chin*, 1999). Despite what might be construed as a good faith effort on the part of the juries in the *James* and *Chin* cases to impress upon health care professionals the ethical imperative to address pain and suffering, the response of the medical profession has been underwhelming. There has been a collective cacophony of weeping, wailing, and gnashing of teeth as physicians lament that they are between a rock and a hard place, subject to regulatory board sanction or possibly even criminal prosecution if they are too liberal in prescribing opioids and subject to civil liability by patients or families if they are too conservative.

Physician-Assisted Suicide and the Pursuit of a Peaceful Death

Another reason that the decade of the 1990s proved to be the crucible for change in pain management and end-of-life care was that the debate over physician-assisted suicide (PAS) moved into both the legislative and judicial arenas. Two pivotal events were the passage (by voter initiative) of the Oregon Death with Dignity Act in 1994 and the decisions by the U.S. Supreme Court in 1997 of companion cases challenging statutes in the states of Washington and New York that made assisting in a suicide a criminal offense. While a unanimous Supreme Court ruled that there is no federal constitutional right to PAS, a majority of the justices, writing in concurring opinions, intimated that there may well be a constitutional liberty interest on the part of dying patients in receiving whatever medications at whatever levels may be necessary to ensure that they do not suffer in their dying. This purported liberty interest would encompass palliative measures that carry a known and significant risk of rendering the patient unconscious and/or hastening the patient's death. (We will return to this point later, when we discuss palliative options of last resort and their moral justification.)

Among the chief arguments of the opponents to PAS was the insistence that virtually all pain and suffering at the end of life could and should be relieved with conventional means that are clinically, ethically, and legally acceptable. Therefore, so the argument runs, there is no need to take the radical step onto the slippery slope of legalizing and regulating PAS for patients with a terminal condition (Foley, 1995). The key words in this analysis are "could" and "should," and the problem with the heavy reliance on them by the opponents of PAS is that the available data did not—and for the most part still do not—support the contention that what is theoretically possible and morally obligatory is, in fact, what is consistently done. The gap is only occasionally between what health care professionals know and what they actually apply in their customary practice; more often, it is between what they should but do not know and how that compromises their ability to assess and manage pain.

THE CULPABILITY OF CULTIVATED IGNORANCE

There is a moral dimension to these pervasive professional knowledge deficits, the implications of which transcend the individual professional and reach the health professions as a whole. The very concept of professionalism presupposes possession of knowledge, skills, and attitudes that are essential to effective practice. Within the ambit of unprofessional conduct is the failure to possess or appropriately apply such knowledge, skills, and attitudes (AMA, 2002). The knowledge deficits of physicians concerning the assessment and management of pain have been documented in the clinical literature since at least the early 1970s, yet persistent calls in that literature for reform in the health professions curricula have been ignored with impunity. Eric Cassell, for example, writes:

> The obligation of physicians to relieve human suffering stretches back into antiquity. Despite this fact, little attention is explicitly given to the problem of suffering in medical education, research, or practice …. My colleagues of a contemplative nature were surprised how little they knew of the problem and how little thought they had given to it, whereas medical students tended to be unsure of the relevance of the issue to their work. (Cassell, 1982, pp. 639-640, 639-640)

This failure or refusal to modify curricula to ensure that graduating health care professionals—in particular, physicians and nurses—possess minimal core competencies in pain assessment and management constitutes the cultivation of ignorance in this area, for which the responsible parties should be culpable. Such culpability is recognized in the law, which traditionally provides that an individual can be held accountable not just for what he or she actually knows but also for what, in the reasonable exercise of due diligence, he or she ought to know. Indeed, this concept of the culpability of cultivated ignorance goes to the very core of the concept of a professional, which is the commitment to lifelong learning.

For further confirmation of the pervasiveness of these knowledge deficits, one need look no further than the American Medical Association's Education for Physicians in End-of-Life Care (EPEC) project, which was developed in the late 1990s through a substantial grant from the Robert Wood Johnson Foundation. The underlying premise for the project was that many, perhaps even most, physicians graduate from medical school and residency training programs without the core competencies essential to providing minimally sufficient care to patients at the end of life. The goal of EPEC was to develop a far-flung cadre of physicians (through an extensive series of train-the-trainer seminars) who would widely disseminate the EPEC materials to their colleagues, as well as serve as role models and mentors in health care institutions throughout the country. A related project has been developed and disseminated for nurses as the End-of-Life Nursing Education Consortium (ELNEC).

OPIOPHOBIA AND THE CULTURE OF PAIN

As a society, however, we must acknowledge that there are barriers to health care professionals' consistently and conscientiously applying such knowledge and skills, even when they do possess them. These barriers to the relief of pain and suffering have primarily to do with fears of a legal nature and are directly linked to past patterns and practices of professional licensing organizations and the Federal Drug Enforcement Administration (DEA) in the area of prescribing and administering controlled substances.

During the latter decades of the 20th century, when studies indicated that the United States was experiencing an epidemic of undertreated pain, state medical licensing boards were routinely initiating disciplinary actions against physicians for so-called "overprescribing" of opioid analgesics; meanwhile, the concept of "underprescribing" (i.e., failing or refusing to provide necessary or appropriate analgesia) was altogether unheard of in medical board practice. This practice of taking draconian disciplinary action against physicians who dared to aggressively manage the pain of their patients led to the anomalous state of affairs in which health care professionals were required to engage in acts of moral courage simply to ensure that their patients with moderate-to-severe pain did not suffer unnecessarily (*Hoover v. Agency for Health Care Administration*, 1996). Physicians who knew that they were providing less analgesia (weaker medications or lower doses) than their patients' conditions required for effective pain management sought to exempt themselves from moral responsibility by contending that it was not unreasonable for them to practice a form of "defensive medicine" that was necessary to keep their prescribing practices below the radar screen of the regulators. This attitude, however, runs directly counter to the fundamental nature of the fiduciary duty health care professionals owe to their patients, which is to act only in the pursuit of the patient's interests and well-being and not their own.

Palliative Options of Last Resort

To fully understand and appreciate the ethical implications of the interventions commonly considered to be "palliative options of last resort," one must be able to conceive of a medical fate worse than death. Individuals, including health care professionals, whose powers of empathy and imagination or whose religious convictions make it impossible to entertain such a conception will be likely to reject any ethical justification for the use of any of these options. However, given the current clinical fact—which is that some terminal patients experience significant pain, suffering, and distress caused by refractory symptoms—we can only hope that these professionals will not gravitate toward settings in which they are likely to encounter dying patients. The critical issue is not whether the clinician believes that the patient's condition meets the conditions for a fate worse than death, but whether the patient does. If so, there is a moral obligation and professional responsibility to offer one or more options so as not to abandon the patient to his or her suffering (Quill & Cassel, 1995).

One commonly mentioned option is for a patient with decisional capacity to voluntarily stop eating and drinking (VSED). Patients who exercise this option typically do so because they believe that the burdens of continuing to live until death comes from the natural progression of their underlying condition so far outweigh any benefits that an earlier death (most likely from dehydration) is preferable. However, during the weeks that it will take for the patient to die once VSED is undertaken, the patient is likely to require other aggressive palliative measures, depending on the nature of his or her diagnosis, symptoms, and experience of illness (Printz, 1992).

Throughout the debates over the legitimacy of PAS as a palliative option of last resort, the most frequently mentioned alternative for the relief of intractable pain and suffering or refractory symptoms associated with terminal illness is terminal sedation. The supporters of terminal sedation assiduously maintain that clinically, ethically, and legally it is different from PAS. Not surprisingly, its critics maintain otherwise (Orentlicher, 1997). Precision in the use of terminology is critical to sound ethical analysis, but particularly so in emotionally and politically charged issues such as these. We, therefore, begin with a definition, description, and conceptual analysis of terminal sedation, including the articulation of important distinctions among terminal sedation and two closely related terms: total sedation and conscious sedation.

Terminal sedation involves two separate elements; separating these two elements will enable us to distinguish between terminal sedation and the closely related approach of total sedation. *Terminal sedation* involves the total sedation of the patient and the withholding of artificial nutrition and hydration (ANH) for patients who, prior to sedation, could take these by mouth or the withdrawing of ANH from patients who were previously receiving it. *Total sedation*, in contrast, involves only the first element—sedation to unconsciousness in response to otherwise intractable pain or refractory symptoms—but with the initiation or continuation of ANH. Total sedation is the less controversial of the two approaches because, when it is properly administered and the patient is appropriately monitored and managed, the patient's subsequent demise is generally considered to be the result of the underlying terminal illness-neither caused by nor contributed to by the sedation process. This proposition is not without its critics, however, given the increased risks of life-threatening side effects associated with the use of barbiturates to induce and maintain heavy sedation (Truog, Berde, Mitchell, & Grier, 1992). *Conscious sedation* seeks to relieve anxiety, enable patient cooperation, and produce some amnesia. Even when maintained for weeks or longer, it poses fewer risks but may not be sufficient to ensure adequate relief in difficult cases at the end of life (Rousseau, 1996).

When ANH are withheld or withdrawn as an integral component of terminal sedation, it becomes considerably more difficult to persuasively maintain that the patient's subsequent demise was the result of the natural progression of the underlying disease process rather than from dehydration, just as a patient who elects (VSED) is considered to be consciously and deliberately choosing to hasten death. The moral and religious debate over nutrition and hydration in the gravely or terminally ill has been jolted from a state of relative torpor by the recent high-profile case of Terri Schiavo. Although a permanent vegetative state (PVS) has a prognosis that strongly suggests that the patient will not survive to his or her natural lifespan, even with excellent care, the common perception was that the cause of Schiavo's death was dehydration, not complications from a PVS (Brown, 2005).

The renewed attention to ANH compels us to take a closer look at the rationale most commonly offered for why terminal and total sedation are morally acceptable palliative options of last resort but PAS is not. We begin with an important observation made by Justice Sandra Day O'Connor in her concurring opinion in the *Cruzan* case, in which the parents of Nancy Cruzan, who had been in a PVS for several years, sought to have her ANH discontinued. O'Connor observed that, contrary to the assertions by the State of Missouri, which opposed its withdrawal, ANH is an invasive medical procedure (as opposed to the mere provision of food and water) that requires informed consent either by the patient or the patient's proxy, both initially and on a continuing basis (*Cruzan v. Director, Missouri Department of Health*, 1990).

The argument in support of the ethical propriety of terminal sedation typically takes the following form. The patient, or the patient's proxy, has determined that pain and/or symptom management of a kind and at a level that preserves the patient's consciousness is inadequate to alleviate the patient's suffering. Total sedation will ensure that the patient does not suffer. Because the patient is in the advanced stages of a terminal illness and there is no reason to believe that the patient will ever again be conscious, ANS provides the patient with no medical benefit and, therefore, may reasonably be withheld with the prior consent of the patient or proxy. The physician's intent (which is considered to be crucial in assessing the morality of his or her actions) in providing total sedation is to alleviate otherwise intractable suffering. Furthermore, the intent in withholding (or, in some cases, withdrawing) ANH is either to respect the patient's autonomous choice (or that of the patient's proxy) or to allow a natural death by refraining from prolonging the dying process with an invasive medical procedure that can no longer confer medical benefit on the patient.

The phraseology "allowing natural death" has acquired an increased following of late and has been offered as a reasonable alternative to "Do Not Resuscitate" orders, which are considered to erroneously convey a form of patient abandonment. The term draws on a once common but now largely discredited moral distinction between actively and passively participating in a patient's death. The foundation for the active-passive distinction was never strong, particularly when it was used to justify on moral grounds withdrawing life-sustaining therapies (LSTs) while at the same time morally critiquing PAS. As a matter of logic and common sense, extubating a mechanically ventilated patient or removing a surgically implanted gastrostomy tube seems much more "active" (and makes the clinician much more involved in bringing about the patient's death) than writing a prescription for a lethal dose of medication that the patient may then ingest (Quill, Lo, & Brock, 1997).

The arguments in support of withdrawing LSTs and against PAS were based on two additional factors. First, the clinician's intent in withdrawing LSTs is to respect the wishes (and hence the autonomy) of the patient. Second, the cause of a patient's death following withdrawal of an LST is considered to be the underlying disease, not the clinician's action in discontinuing the LST. In writing a lethal prescription (so the argument continues), the clinician's intent must necessarily be to provide the means for the patient to hasten death, and any death that results from ingestion of a lethal prescription must be from the medication and not from the underlying terminal condition.

The argument in support of PAS is that the clinician's intent in writing the prescription can be every bit as much about respecting the autonomous choice of the patient as the withdrawal of life support. Furthermore, it is fallacious to maintain that a ventilator-dependent patient who is extubated dies from the underlying medical condition rather than from the direct and immediate sequelae of extubation (Beauchamp & Childress, 1994). A similar argument can be made with regard to the cause of death of a terminally sedated patient. The patient dies of dehydration, not of the underlying terminal condition that caused the suffering that necessitated complete sedation. It is important to note that arguments such as these are not made to establish the impropriety of withdrawing LSTs or providing terminal sedation but rather to establish that PAS as practiced in Oregon is also appropriate when the requirements of the Oregon Death with Dignity Act have been met.

DOCTRINE OF DOUBLE EFFECT

As the previous discussion shows, the intent of the clinician is crucial to an adequate ethical analysis of his or her conduct in the care of a dying patient. However, "intent" is a subjective state of mind of the actor about which no one else has direct, immediate, and authoritative knowledge. Intent also plays a crucial role in a medieval approach to ethical analysis, the Doctrine of Double Effect (DDE), which has gained a remarkable prominence in contemporary debates over issues of end-of-life care.

DDE is believed to have originated in the thought and writings of the medieval philosopher and theologian Thomas Aquinas. The purpose of DDE is to provide a basis on which to assess the ultimate ethical propriety of an action that has both good and bad consequences. DDE has four essential features or conditions, each of which must be fulfilled in order for an action to be deemed morally acceptable (Quinn, 1989):

- The action itself must be either morally good or morally neutral.
- The bad result must not be directly intended (in contradistinction to foreseen).
- The good result must not be proximately caused by the bad result.
- The good result must be proportionate to the bad result.

A quintessential example of the application of DDE to a contemporary ethical controversy is the administration of increasing doses of opioid analgesics to dying patients in an effort to ensure that they do not suffer in their dying. The action itself is deemed morally good because of the clinician's well-recognized responsibility to relieve suffering. The specific intent of the clinician is to relieve suffering, although there is known risk of respiratory depression. The good result is the relief of pain and suffering, and it is not achieved by hastening the patient's death, even though that may occur. Finally, the relief of suffering is considered to be proportionate to the risk of a hastened death in a patient with advanced terminal illness (AHCPR, 1994).

The U.S. Supreme Court implicitly relied on DDE when it discussed the currently available alternatives to PAS. The critical language appears in a concurring opinion by Justice O'Connor:

…a patient who is suffering from a terminal illness and who is experiencing great pain has no legal barriers to obtaining medication, from qualified physicians, to alleviate that suffering, even to the point of causing unconsciousness and hastening death. (*Washington v. Glucksberg*, 1997)

The problem, which O'Connor's assertion fails to acknowledge, is that there is nothing more than a reasonable inference that the physician's intent in prescribing increasing doses of opioids is to ensure effective palliation. Were a terminal patient to die shortly after administration of an increased dose of morphine, the Supreme Court's apparent acceptance of DDE would not prevent a distressed family member of the patient or an overzealous prosecutor from taking legal action against the clinician based on the well-established legal principle that every person may be presumed to intend the natural and probable consequences of his or her actions. Under this principle, the clinician knew (or should have known) what would happen and, therefore, may be presumed to have intended to hasten the patient's death rather than to relieve his or her symptoms (Nuccetelli & Seay, 2000). In recent years, a limited number of physicians have been criminally prosecuted on facts similar to these, with mixed results (Alpers, 1998).

DDE is not without its critics on philosophical grounds as well (Quill, Brock, & Dresser, 1997). DDE presupposes that there will be at least a strong consensus, if not unanimity, on fundamental points such as whether the act under consideration is morally good or neutral and whether the good result is commensurate with the bad. One need only consider the profound moral disagreements Americans have over the ethical propriety of PAS, withdrawing ANH from patients like Terri Schiavo, and conducting human embryonic stem cell research to realize how elusive such consensus can be.

CONCLUSION

Hard-line positions that purport to distinguish the clearly ethical from the clearly unethical, and their civil and criminal law corollaries, do not ultimately advance the cause of improving end-of-life care. There is no safe harbor from which clinicians may provide competent and compassionate care of the dying and remain completely protected from the vicissitudes of public opinion, social policy, and the personal agendas of those who seek to shape one or both of these to their own ends. Fortunately, there are now many state and national guidelines and policies pertaining to all aspects of end-of-life care. If clinicians use these resources in a good faith effort to provide competent and compassionate care, they and their patients will be well served. When the process of dying entails rigors that render consciousness unbearable, what patients often wish has been captured elegantly and powerfully by Joseph Conrad in his classic novel *Lord Jim*:

> He might have been resigned to die, but I suspect he wanted to die without added terrors, quietly, in a sort of peaceful trance. A certain readiness to perish is not so very rare, but it is seldom that you meet men whose souls, steeled in the impenetrable armor of resolution, are ready to fight a losing battle to the last. The desire for peace waxes stronger as hope declines, until at last it conquers the very desire of life. Who of us has not observed this, or perhaps experienced something of that feeling in his own person—this extreme weariness of emotions, the vanity of effort, the yearning for rest. (Conrad, 1986, p. 108) ■

Ben A. Rich, JD, PhD, is associate professor of bioethics at the University of California, Davis School of Medicine, with appointments in the Departments of Internal Medicine and Anesthesiology and Pain Medicine. He is editor of the Forensic Pain Medicine Section of the journal Pain Medicine, and a member of the Council of Ethics of the American Academy of Pain Medicine and the Ethics Committee of the American College of Legal Medicine. He has published extensively in academic and professional journals on ethical and legal issues in pain management and end-of-life care, and is the author of the book Strange Bedfellows: How Medical Jurisprudence Has Influenced Medical Ethics and Medical Practice *(KluwerAcademic/Plenum Press, 2001).*

REFERENCES

Agency for Health Care Policy and Research. (1994). *Management of cancer pain.* Washington, DC: Department of Health and Human Services.

Alpers, A. (1998). Criminal act or palliative care: Prosecutions involving the care of the dying. *Journal of Law, Medicine and Ethics, 26*, 308-331.

American Medical Association. (2002). *Code of medical ethics.* Chicago: AMA.

Beauchamp, T. L., & Childress, J. T. (1994). *Principles of biomedical ethics* (4th ed.). New York: Oxford University Press.

Bergman v. Chin, No. H205732-1, Cal. Dept. Sup. Ct. (Feb. 16, 1999).

Brown, D. (2005, March 23). Little known about starvation death. *Washington Post*, p. A5.

Cassell, E. J. (1982). The nature of suffering and the goals of medicine. *New England Journal of Medicine, 306*, 639-640.

Conrad, J. (1986). *Lord Jim.* London: Penguin Books, p. 108.

Cruzan v. Director, Missouri Department of Health, 497 U.S. 261 (1990).

Cushing, M. (1992). Pain management on trial. *American Journal of Nursing, 92*, 21-23.

Estate of Henry James v. Hillhaven Corporation, No. 89 CVS 64, N.C. Sup. Ct. (Jan. 15, 1991).

Foley, K. M. (1995). Pain, physician-assisted suicide, and euthanasia. *Pain Forum, 4*, 163-178.

Hoover v. Agency for Health Care Administration, 676 So. 2d 1380, Fla. Dist. Ct. App. (1996).

Melzack, R. (1990). The tragedy of needless pain. *Scientific American, 262*, 27-33.

Morris, D. B. (1991). *The culture of pain.* Berkeley, CA: University of California Press.

Nuccetelli, S., & Seay, G. (2000). Relieving pain and foreseeing death: A paradox about accountability and blame. *Journal of Law, Medicine and Ethics, 28*, 19-24.

Orentlicher, D. (1997). The Supreme Court and physician-assisted suicide: Rejecting assisted suicide but embracing euthanasia. *New England Journal of Medicine, 337*, 1237-1239.

Printz, L. A. (1992). Terminal dehydration, a compassionate treatment. *Archives of Internal Medicine, 152*, 697-700.

Quill, T. E., Brock, D. W., & Dresser, R. (1997). The rule of double effect: A critique of its role in end-of-life decision making. *New England Journal of Medicine, 337*, 1768-1771.

Quill, T. E., & Cassel, C. K. (1995). Nonabandonment: A central obligation for physicians. *Annals of Internal Medicine, 122*, 368-374.

Quill, T. E., Lo, B., & Brock, D. W. (1997). Palliative options of last resort: A comparison of voluntarily stopping eating and drinking, terminal sedation, physician-assisted suicide, and voluntary active euthanasia. *Journal of the American Medical Association, 278*, 2099-2104.

Quinn, W. S. (1989). Actions, intentions, and consequences: The doctrine of double effect. *Philosophy and Public Affairs, 18*, 334-351.

Rousseau, P. (1996). Terminal sedation in the care of dying patients. *Archives of Internal Medicine, 156*, 1785-1786.

Truog, R. D., Berde, C. B., Mitchell, C., & Grier, H. E. (1992). Barbiturates in the care of the terminally ill. *New England Journal of Medicine, 327*, 1678-1682.

Wanzer, S. H., Federman, D. D., Adelstein, S. J., Cassel, C. K., Cassem, E. H., Cranford, R. E., et al. (1989). The physician's responsibility toward hopelessly ill patients: A second look. *New England Journal of Medicine, 320*, 844-849.

Washington v. Glucksberg, 521 U.S. 702 (1997).

SELF-ASSESSMENT OF PAIN

No one knows your pain more than you so you have an important role in assessing your pain. These questions may help you in describing your pain to health care professionals.

- On a scale of 0 to 10 (with 0 as no pain and 10 as unbearable pain), how much pain are you experiencing now? What is the "best" the pain becomes? What is the worst?

- Do you notice any times during the day that the pain develops, increases, or decreases? For example, how does pain relate to activities such as eating, sleeping, or taking medications? Do any activities or procedures seem to cause, increase, or decrease your pain?

- How does the pain interfere with your daily functioning? Are there activities that you can no longer do because of the pain? Are other activities more difficult because of the pain?

- How do you experience the pain? Is it a dull ache, sharp pains, or a burning sensation? Is it localized—occurring in one area—or felt throughout the body? Do you have different experiences of pain throughout the day?

- What do you do to relieve pain once you experience it? Do you take any medication (prescribed, over-the-counter, or other medication)? Are there any folk remedies that you use? Do you change your behavior in any way— sitting, breathing, or resting, for example? Do these actions help? If they do, how long does that relief generally last?

You remain your best health care advocate. By carefully observing your own pain, you can assist health professionals in managing and treating that pain.

CHAPTER 15

Resources

Lisa McGahey Veglahn

American Academy of Hospice and Palliative Medicine
4700 W. Lake Avenue
Glenview, IL 60025-1485
(847) 375-4712
www.aahpm.org
info@aahpm.org

The American Academy of Hospice and Palliative Medicine (AAHPM) is an organization of physicians and other medical professionals dedicated to excellence in and advancement of palliative medicine through prevention and relief of patient and family suffering by providing education and clinical practice standards, fostering research, facilitating personal and professional development, and by public policy advocacy. The Web site includes a section of End of Life/Palliative Care Educational Resources to search peer-reviewed resources and to submit new materials.

American Academy of Pain Management
13947 Mono Way, #A
Sonora, CA 95370
(209) 533-9744
www.aapainmanage.org
aapm@aapainmanage.org

The American Academy of Pain Management is the largest pain organization in the United States. It provides credentialing, accreditation of facilities, networking opportunities, continuing education, quality publications, and an annual clinical meeting. Its goal is to bring together the many professionals who work with individuals in pain and to assist in the creation of quality services for those individuals.

American Alliance of Cancer Pain Initiatives

AACPI c/o University of Wisconsin Medical School
Rm. 4720, 1300 University Avenue
Madison, WI 53706
(608) 265-4013
www.aacpi.wisc.edu
aacpi@mailplus.wisc.edu

The American Alliance of Cancer Pain Initiatives (AACPI) is dedicated to promoting cancer pain relief nationwide by supporting the efforts of State Cancer Pain Initiatives—voluntary, grassroots organizations that provide education and advocacy to health care providers, cancer patients, and their families. The AACPI provides national leadership and advocacy for the Initiative movement, recommends program direction, supports Initiative growth and development, and fosters collaborations with other organizations. The Resource Center of the AACPI (http://wiscinfo.doit.wisc.edu/trc/) is dedicated to improving pain management nationwide by supporting the work of the State Cancer Pain Initiatives and by developing programs and educational resources to positively influence health care systems, the regulatory climate, and the culture at large.

American Pain Foundation

201 North Charles Street, Suite 710
Baltimore, MD 21201-4111
(888) 615-PAIN (7246)
www.painfoundation.org
info@painfoundation.org

The American Pain Foundation is an independent nonprofit organization serving people with pain through information, advocacy, and support. Its mission is to improve the quality of life of people with pain by raising public awareness, providing practical information, promoting research, and advocating to remove barriers and increase access to effective pain management. Its Web site includes a disease-specific links page and will soon feature an online discussion board with a broad range of topics relating to pain and end-of-life care.

American Pain Society
4700 W. Lake Avenue
Glenview, IL 60025
(847) 375-4715
www.ampainsoc.org
info@ampainsoc.org

The mission of the American Pain Society (APS) is to advance pain-related research, education, treatment, and professional practice. As the leading professional society in the field of pain management, the American Pain Society supports the congressional mandate declaring 2000-2010 the Decade of Pain Control and Research (www.decadeofpain.org). APS believes the key to better understanding pain and treating it most effectively is through pain research and increased professional and public understanding of pain and pain management. APS is one of several pain organizations developing professional and public awareness programs in conjunction with the Decade of Pain Control and Research. (See Decade of Pain under Web Sites for more information.) APS's Web site includes a Position Statement on Treatment of Pain at the End of Life.

**APPEAL: A Progressive Palliative Care Educational Curriculum
for the Care of African Americans at Life's End**
PO Box 5911
Hyattsville, MD 20782
(301) 559-3492
www.appealproject.org
info@appealproject.org

The purpose of the APPEAL project is to educate health care professionals on essential clinical competencies and practical skills needed to provide culturally appropriate, palliative, and quality end-of-life care services to African-American patients and their families. The initial goal of APPEAL is to expand upon and enhance other curricula that have covered relevant aspects of end-of-life care and decision making for physicians and health care providers by recognizing and addressing barriers to care, disparity issues, access to quality care, and the cultural needs, traditions, and preferences of African-American patients and family members.

Association for Death Education and Counseling

60 Revere Drive, Suite 500
Northbrook, IL 60062
(847) 509-0403
www.adec.org
adec@adec.org

The Association for Death Education and Counseling is an international professional organization dedicated to promoting excellence in death education, care of the dying, and bereavement counseling and support. Based on quality research and theory, the association provides information, support, and resources to its multicultural, multidisciplinary membership and, through it, to the public.

Compassion & Choices

PO Box 101810
Denver, CO 80250-1810
(800) 247-7421
www.compassionandchoices.org
info@compassionandchoices.org

Created in 2005 by the unification of Compassion in Dying and End-of-Life Choices, Compassion & Choices supports, educates, and advocates for choice and care at the end of life. Compassion & Choices works for improved care and expanded options at the end of life, with effective care for every dying person. Compassion & Choices supports comprehensive pain control and palliative care.

The Foundation for End-of-Life Care

100 South Biscayne Boulevard, Suite 1500
Miami, FL 33131
(877) 800-2951 or (305) 350-6978
www.vitascharityfund.org

The Foundation for End-of-Life Care, a not-for-profit organization established by VITAS Healthcare Corporation, was created to improve end-of-life care for individual patients and their families while supporting fundamental societal change. The foundation provides resources to advance the quality of end-of-life care through support of the Duke Institute on Care at the End of Life, as well as through research grants, partnerships, and individual grants.

Intercultural Cancer Center
Intercultural Cancer Council
6655 Travis, Suite 322
Houston, TX 77030
(713) 798-4617
www.iccnetwork.org
info@iccnetwork.org

The Intercultural Cancer Council (ICC) promotes policies, programs, partnerships, and research to eliminate the unequal burden of cancer among racial and ethnic minorities and medically underserved populations in the United States and its associated territories. The ICC provides downloadable fact sheets on subjects such as pain and cancer.

National Association of Attorneys General—
End-of-Life Health Care Project
750 First Street, NE, Suite 1100
Washington, DC 20002
(202) 326-6000
www.naag.org/issues/issue-endoflife.php

The National Association of Attorneys General (NAAG) End-of-Life Health Care project is now acting as a clearinghouse for the state Attorneys General offices. The project was begun by Oklahoma Attorney General Drew Edmondson when he was president of the National Association of Attorneys General; his vision has encouraged many Attorneys General offices to become even more actively engaged in helping to improve end-of-life care for the citizens of their states. The NAAG End-of-Life Health Care Project has focused on three principal areas in which Attorneys General may play a major role: pain management, acknowledgment, and respect for the wishes of those who are dying, and ensuring competent end-of-life care.

National Association of Social Workers

750 First Street, NE, Suite 700

Washington, DC 20002-4241

(202) 408-8600

www.naswdc.org

membership@naswdc.org

The National Association of Social Workers (NASW) is the largest membership organization of professional social workers in the world, with 153,000 members. NASW works to enhance the professional growth and development of its members, to create and maintain professional standards, and to advance sound social policies.

National Hospice and Palliative Care Organization

1700 Diagonal Road, Suite 625

Alexandria, VA 22314

(703) 837-1500

Consumer HelpLine: (800) 658-8898

www.nhpco.org

nhpco_info@nhpco.org

The National Hospice and Palliative Care Organization (NHPCO) is the largest nonprofit membership organization representing hospice and palliative care programs and professionals in the United States. The organization is committed to improving end-of-life care and expanding access to hospice. NHPCO offers educational programs and materials for professionals and the public.

Pain and Policy Studies Group

406 Science Drive, Suite 202

Madison, WI 53711-1068

(608) 263-7662

www.medsch.wisc.edu/painpolicy/index.htm

ppsg@med.wisc.edu

The mission of the Pain and Policy Studies Group (PPSG) is to "balance" international, national, and state policies to ensure adequate availability of pain medications for patient care while minimizing diversion and abuse, and to support a global communications program to improve access to information about pain relief, palliative care, and policy. The purpose of the PPSG Web site, which includes material published by the PPSG and other authoritative sources, is to facilitate public access to information about pain relief and public policy. The Pain & Policy Studies Group at the University of Wisconsin addresses both domestic and international policy issues and is a World Health Organization Collaborating Center for Policy and Communications in Cancer Care.

Partners for Understanding Pain

www.theacpa.org/pu_main.asp

Partners for Understanding Pain is a loose consortium of organizations with an interest in the personal, economic, and social impact of pain on our society. Members include health-condition-specific groups as well as those with broader mandates that touch the lives of people with chronic, acute, and cancer pain. The partners' mission is to create greater understanding among health care professionals, individuals, and families who are struggling with pain management, the business community, legislators, and the general public that pain is a serious public health issue; offer a comprehensive network of resources and knowledge about issues in pain management through the members, each of which brings its unique perspective to the dialogue; and build understanding and support that can help people with chronic, acute, and cancer pain lead better lives. Purdue Pharma LP is a Gold Level Sponsor of Partners for Understanding Pain.

WEB SITES

Cancer-pain.org

www.cancer-pain.org

Cancer-pain.org has been developed by the Association of Cancer Online Resources with input and advice from patients, caregivers, and an advisory board of health care professionals dedicated to providing the most advanced cancer pain relief. The aim is to help cancer patients receive the pain treatment they deserve. The site offers in-depth information to assist in pain management decision making and interactive discussion groups to help patients determine what will work for them.

Child Cancer Pain

www.childcancerpain.org/home.cfm

Sponsored by the Texas Cancer Council (www.txcancer.org), this Web site serves as a resource, focused on pain management, for health professionals who care for children with cancer. A better understanding of the nature of pain, new interventions, agents, and methods of pain medication delivery are essential components to improving a child's care and quality of life. The site offers continuing education credit for those who complete the requirements.

Decade of Pain

www.decadeofpain.org

The American Pain Society (APS) supports the congressional mandate declaring 2000-2010 as the Decade of Pain Control and Research. This Web site provides helpful information on related pain initiatives, current events in pain management, and other opportunities for advancing support for optimal pain management in the United States. APS is one of several pain organizations developing professional and public awareness programs in conjunction with the Decade of Pain Control and Research.

End of Life/Palliative Education Resource Center

www.eperc.mcw.edu

The purpose of the End of Life/Palliative Education Resource Center is to share educational resource material among the community of health professional educators involved in palliative care education. The site includes education materials, downloadable fast facts, and a "Starter Kit" of preselected articles, books, teaching materials, and Web resources that have been assembled for beginners—medical educators who have recently accepted a new teaching role, have been asked to build a curriculum, or have decided to become Board Certified in Hospice and Palliative Medicine.

Growthhouse

www.growthhouse.org

info@growthhouse.org

Growth House, Inc., serves as a portal to resources for life-threatening illness and end-of-life care. Its primary mission is to improve the quality of compassionate care for people who are dying through public education and global professional collaboration. The Web site has an excellent search engine that offers access to the Internet's most comprehensive collection of reviewed resources for end-of-life care. It also hosts an online Professional Forum on Pain and Symptom Management in Terminal Care.

The Mayday Pain Project

www.painandhealth.org

The major goal of the Mayday Pain Project is to increase awareness and provide objective information concerning the treatment of pain. The Web site, which is set up to be an index for visitors, contains carefully chosen Internet links and resources for use by everyone from pain sufferers to family members and caregivers to medical professionals.

MedLinePlus

www.medlineplus.gov/

MedLinePlus is a service of the National Library of Medicine, the National Institutes of Health, and other government agencies and health-related organizations. MEDLINE searches are included in MedLinePlus and give easy access to medical journal articles. MedLinePlus also has a dictionary, an illustrated medical encyclopedia, and the latest health news.

Pain.com

www.pain.com

Pain.com strives to be the premier educational and informational resource on the Internet for health care professionals and consumers who have an interest in pain and its management. Supported by the Dannemiller Memorial Educational Foundation, Pain.com provides free medical educational and informational content. By providing a variety of accredited activities for physicians, pharmacists, and nurses, the Dannemiller Memorial Educational Foundation seeks to foster an environment where health care professionals can grow in their knowledge and management of pain. The Dannemiller Memorial Educational Foundation further seeks to empower pain sufferers and their caregivers with information to better equip them to work in partnership with their physician to actively manage their pain.

PainEDU.org
www.painedu.org

PainEDU.org is a resource for clinically relevant information about pain assessment and management. PainEDU.org offers medical professionals the opportunity to stay current with news and literature in the pain management field, to meet some of the leading pain practitioners, and to earn continuing education credits.

Pain and the Law
www.painandthelaw.org

This site has been developed by the Center for Health Law Studies at Saint Louis University and the American Society of Law, Medicine and Ethics under a grant from the Mayday Fund. The site includes information on palliative medicine.

The Palliative Cancer Education Section of the American Association for Cancer Education
www.cancer-research.umaryland.edu/pc-web.htm

The Palliative Cancer Education Section of the American Association for Cancer Education (www.aaceonline.com) is dedicated to advancing all areas of palliative medicine education, including, but not limited to, pain and symptom management, end-of-life communication, breaking bad news, psychosocial and spiritual aspects, medical ethics, and medical legal issues.

StopPain.org
www.stoppain.org

This Web site is run by the Department of Pain Medicine and Palliative Care at Beth Israel Medical Center. The Web site offers a comprehensive pain glossary for professionals and consumers.

SPECIALTY-SPECIFIC PROFESSIONAL ORGANIZATIONS

The American Academy of Pain Medicine

4700 W. Lake Avenue
Glenview, IL 60025
(847) 375-4731
www.painmed.org
aapm@amtec.com

The American Academy of Pain Medicine (AAPM) is the medical specialty society representing physicians practicing in the field of pain medicine. As a medical specialty society, AAPM is involved in education, training, advocacy, and research in the specialty of pain medicine. Its mission is to promote quality care of patients with pain as a symptom of disease and primary pain disease through research, education, and advocacy, and through advancement of the specialty of pain medicine.

The American Medical Directors Association

10480 Little Patuxent Parkway, Suite 760
Columbia, MD 21044
(410) 740-9743 OR (800) 876-2632 toll-free
www.amda.com
webmaster@amda.com

The American Medical Directors Association (AMDA) is the professional association of medical directors and physicians practicing in the long-term care continuum, dedicated to excellence in patient care by providing education, advocacy, information, and professional development. AMDA's Web site includes clinical practice guidelines on pain management in the long-term care setting and other resources.

American Society for Pain Management Nursing
PO Box 15473
Lenexa, KS 66285-5473
(888) 34A-SPMN or (913) 752-4975
www.aspmn.org
aspmn@goamp.com

The mission of the American Society for Pain Management Nursing (ASPMN) is to advance and promote optimal nursing care for people affected by pain. ASPMN's goals include enhancing access to quality care, raising public awareness about pain management, and providing professional resources.

Education for Physicians on End-of-Life Care Project
The EPEC Project
Northwestern University, Feinberg School of Medicine
750 N. Lake Shore Drive, Suite 601
Chicago, IL 60611
(312) 503-EPEC
www.epec.net
info@epec.net

EPEC's mission is to educate all health care professionals on the essential clinical competencies in palliative care. Programs include train the trainer workshops, national meetings, and online learning. The *EPEC Curriculum* combines didactic sessions, videotape presentations, interactive discussions, and practical exercises. It teaches fundamental palliative care skills in communication, ethical decision making, psychosocial considerations, and symptom management. The materials and their take-home messages can be easily adapted to teach interdisciplinary audiences.

ELNEC (End of Life Nursing Education Consortium)
c/o American Association of Colleges of Nursing
One Dupont Circle, NW, Suite 530
Washington, DC 20036
(202) 463-6930
www.aacn.nche.edu/elnec
pmalloy@aacn.nche.edu

The ELNEC core curriculum is administered by the American Association of Colleges of Nursing. It was developed to prepare qualified nurse educators to provide end-of-life education for nursing students and practicing nurses, and to provide resources to facilitate that instruction. These educators in turn will use the curriculum to integrate end-of-life content for students into undergraduate nursing programs, and offer staff development/continuing education programs for clinical nurses who provide end-of-life care.

Hospice and Palliative Nurses Association
One Penn Center West, Suite 229
Pittsburgh, PA 15276-0100
(412) 787-9301
www.hpna.org
hpna@hpna.org

The purpose of the Hospice and Palliative Nurses Association is to exchange information, experiences, and ideas; to promote understanding of the specialties of hospice and palliative nursing; and to study and promote hospice and palliative nursing research.

■ INDEX ■